Abderrezak BOUAMRA

Advanced Statistical Analysis with SPSS

Abderrezak BOUAMRA

Advanced Statistical Analysis with SPSS

A step-by-step guide

ScienciaScripts

Imprint
Any brand names and product names mentioned in this book are subject to trademark, brand or patent protection and are trademarks or registered trademarks of their respective holders. The use of brand names, product names, common names, trade names, product descriptions etc. even without a particular marking in this work is in no way to be construed to mean that such names may be regarded as unrestricted in respect of trademark and brand protection legislation and could thus be used by anyone.

Cover image: www.ingimage.com

This book is a translation from the original published under ISBN 978-620-3-45400-0.

Publisher:
Sciencia Scripts
is a trademark of
Dodo Books Indian Ocean Ltd. and OmniScriptum S.R.L publishing group

120 High Road, East Finchley, London, N2 9ED, United Kingdom
Str. Armeneasca 28/1, office 1, Chisinau MD-2012, Republic of Moldova, Europe
Printed at: see last page
ISBN: 978-620-6-54281-0

Contents

Preface

After publishing the tomel and tome 2 of data analysis on SPSS software, we are going to present yet another work, this time detailing the various advanced analysis techniques on SPSS software,

In this book, we will explain the various advanced techniques for processing data using SPSS software,

We begin this book with logistic regression, poisson regression, linear regression, the regression equation, MANOVA and multivariate analysis.

For each technique, we illustrate an example by showing the different steps to be followed in SPSS.

We hope to bring back a valuable tool that will enable learners to find solutions to different databases.

I. Logistic regression

1. Problem situation

Logistic regression is a predictive technique commonly used in epidemiology. The aim is to create a model to explain the values taken by a qualitative variable, which is generally binary. This is known as binary logistic regression.

It measures the association between the occurrence of an event (qualitative explained variable) and the factors likely to influence it (explanatory variables). Its main power is to concurrently control the confounding effect between a binary or explained dependent variable and a number of potential risk factors called independent variables.

At present, knowledge of this model and the interpretation of its results have become essential for any medical scientist wishing to develop a more meaningful data analysis. This multiple analysis has become accessible since the arrival of data analysis software.

The aim of this document is not simply to provide the reader with the statistical information needed to carry out logistic regression himself, but also to give him valuable help in understanding the interest of this technique, the basic principles, and above all to provide him with the tools he needs to interpret his results.

2. The benefits of logistic regression

Data analysis in epidemiology often involves detecting a link or relationship between a dependent variable and another independent variable. One difficulty usually encountered is the systematic error in measuring the association between these two variables due to the presence of a third variable called the confounding factor. This confounding bias is usually controllable by adjustment techniques during statistical analysis. However, this Mantel-Haenszel adjustment method is only applicable if the variables are two-class categorical, and to control a single confounding factor. The question is, what should be done if there are several confounders? Is there a statistical adjustment method that can take several confounders into account at the same time?

The advent of statistical software such as SPSS has given us access to new techniques for analysing multivariate data, such as logistic regression, which is capable of controlling all the confounding factors, whatever the type of variable, and quantifying the strength of the association between the event under study and each of the factors influencing it, while taking into account the simultaneous effect of the other factors.

3. Mathematical definition of the logistic regression model

We limit our presentation to a knowledge of the equation of the logistic regression model, and the meaning of its components, knowing that a teacher in medical science does not need to know more details.

The logistics model used is of the form :

$$\text{Logit (y)} = a + B1\ x_{1+}\ B2X_2 + B3X_{33}$$

Y: is the variable to be explained or the dependent variable. The dependent variable is a qualitative dichotomous variable coded (0-1) or (yes/no).

X: is the explanatory variable or the independent variable. This variable could be qualitative or quantitative.

Each variable xi is attached to their coefficients **B**.

Coefficient B (P_i, $_{B2}$, B3   ) which is the logarithm of the odds ratio (OR) associated with each corresponding variable.

Logistic regression can be univariate, but its interest lies in its multivariate application, since it makes it possible to quantify the strength of the link between the variable being explained and each of the explanatory variables, while taking account of the simultaneous effect of all the other explanatory variables included in the model.

In the uni-varied situation the model takes the form :

$$\text{Logit (y)} = a + B1\ x_i$$

4. Which variables should be included in a logistic regression analysis?

In general, the variables that need to be included in a logistic regression analysis are:

- Variables linked to the dependent variable with a probability that chance can explain the occurrence of the event **p < 20%.**
- The risk factors known in the literature are, for example, **smoking** and the occurrence of lung cancer. Smoking is a known risk factor for the disease in the scientific literature.
- The interaction and the two variables in the interaction.
- The matching variable, whether simple matching or frequency matching, has been carried out.

5. Conditions for applying logistic regression

- A linear relationship between the logit (p) of the variable Y and all the quantitative variables X; p value proposes the same approach as for linear regression.
- At least 10 observations for which Y = 0 and Y = 1 for each variable X introduced into the model; if X is a qualitative variable, and N the number of

different possible modalities, this counts as N-1 additional variables.

• It is quite possible, and even frequent, that you will not have a large enough sample size, despite having a large number of observations. This is particularly the case if you have few observations for which Y = 0 or Y = 1, or if you have ordinal categorical variables with a large number of classes.

• The user is therefore invited to reduce the number of explanatory variables if the number of observations is insufficient.

6. Logistic regression methods

Several methods are proposed, and the regression methods available are similar to those for linear regression. However, the selection criterion for progressive methods is different.

You can therefore opt for the **Input** method, and insert all the explanatory variables at the same time. This is the default method proposed and is considered to be the best method, since in this case you will be entering all the explanatory variables yourself and outputting them manually according to the highest score.

This method is particularly useful when you have an interaction. The variables making up this interaction can only be removed from the model once the interaction has been eliminated, which is not possible with the other methods.

In addition, if you prefer to select the order **in** which the variables are **entered,** choose the hierarchical method. The parameters will be calculated for each block of variables.

Among the progressive methods, you can always choose **between the step-by-step ascending method** or the **step-by-step descending method.**

In the bottom-up step-by-step method, you will introduce the variable with the highest score first until no variable has a significant score statistic (i.e. smaller than 0.05).

In the top-down step-by-step method, the opposite occurs, since the first model evaluated contains all the variables and the software removes those that do not contribute significantly to improving the prediction.

These two methods are difficult to use if there is an interaction with these two variables once they have been introduced into the model, since the software is a machine that does not prevent one of the two variables from being removed from the model interaction if it has the highest score.

How to keep a variable from a model or eliminate it, whatever the technique used (input, ascending step-by-step and descending step-by-step):

Several methods are proposed for moving from one saturated model to another.

• **Likelihood ratio**: The likelihood ratio measures the adequacy between the distribution observed on a sample and a probability law supposed to describe the reality of the population from which the sample is drawn.

likelihood-ratio, LR: SPSS retains the variable if the change in LR is significant from one model to another when the variable is removed, indicating that this variable contributes to the quality of the fit.

• **Conditional statistics**: this is a less demanding criterion than LR, so it is preferable to prioritise 1er .

• **Wald statistic**: this time, SPSS removes all variables for which the Wald statistic is less than **0.1**. This method can be used with a small sample. Otherwise, it is preferable to use LR.

The "**likelihood ratio**" method is the most widely used to assess the significant contribution to improving prediction of a model saturated with another model.

7. **Logistic regression on SPSS software**

Application - SPSS procedure

We will focus this step on the most interesting tabs in order to carry out a multivariate analysis (logistic regression).

·   To run a logistic regression, click on **Analyse, Regression, Logistique binaire.**

·   In the first dialog box, **insert the dichotomous dependent variable** in the **dependent box** and the explanatory **variables** in the **co-variables** box.

If you want to insert an interaction term between two predictors, select the two variables in the box on the left and click on the

>a*h>

·   Then choose the regression method (default = Input, step-by-step ascending, descending step by step, etc.   ).

-

·   To carry out the analysis, click on '$^!$ ^{jL} .

·   The I$^{!T>}$ '" J button is used to indicate to SPSS which of the variables submitted are qualitative dichotomous (binary). Simply insert them in the Categorical variables box (qualitative) and keep the contrast Default indicator is.

·   The contrast indicator is therefore to be recommended for choosing the first or last category as the reference mode.

·   **The** Enter **button**, as with many types of analysis, is used to enter the results.

It is possible to record certain information of interest as new variables, such as standardised residuals, forecast probabilities (P(Y) values predicted from equation.

·   **The** opt'ons **button:** keep the default options

a.   Step-by-step probability: includes label points for variable selection in progressive methods. Ideally, the criterion should be kept at 0.05 for adding variables and 0.10 for removing them.

b. **Maximum iterations** (20): represents the maximum number of trials SPSS will use to identify the best possible model from the available variables. This should take no more than 20 trials.

c. Include the constant term in the model: the equation includes the coefficient b_0 , which makes the model a better fit to the data.

The other options available may also be relevant.

d. **Hosmer-Lemeshow goodness of fit**: test to assess whether there is a significant difference between the observed values and the predicted values. Obviously, we prefer this test to be non-significant.

e. **CI for exp(b)**: confidence intervals for the coefficient exp(b).

Example: Our example is taken from the article entitled "La production des enseignants algeriens en medecine et ses determinants au cours de la decennie 2000 - 2009. Revue d'Epidemiologie et de Sante Publique ".

In this example :

• **The chosen regression method :**

o We have opted for the **Entree** method proposed by **default** by the software,

o We started inserting all the explanatory variables at the same time, including **the interaction** and the two **interaction** variables.

o The first model to be evaluated contains all the explanatory variables (p < 20%), hence the name of a complete model or a saturated model.

o At each stage, we removed the variable that did not contribute significantly to improving the prediction by using the likelihood ratio **(LR)**: the variable is kept if the change in the LR is significant when the variable is removed, which indicates that this variable contributes to the quality of the fit by applying the x test^2 to a dl.

o The dependent or explained variable is the **status** variable with two modalities (case = teacher who has published), and control = teacher who has not published,

o Among the factors studied (explanatory variables), **faculty, gender, hospital workload, private practice, access to entire articles from private publishers via the Internet, and the number of teachers, assistants and residents were not differentiating factors between cases and controls at the end of the bivariate analysis (p > 0.20)** (see study results).

o All these variables were eliminated using uni-variate analysis.

o Analysis of three-variable tables, each with its own status and two categories (cases and witnesses), revealed **an interaction** between **foreign collaboration** and **collaboration with a biostatistician** and/or epidemiologist (Breslow index test, p = 0.045).

o This interaction was introduced into the multivariate analysis model along with all the variables for which the analysis was pursued with the exception **of age, teaching grade and head of department**.

o Some authors recommend moving directly from univariate analysis to multivariate analysis, without going through the tri-variate analysis stage.

o The importance of this step has been demonstrated in order to highlight an interaction, but also to avoid the effect of redundancy between two variables and therefore facilitate multivariate analysis.

o Age and seniority are redundant variables (85.9% of teachers aged over 50 have more than 15 years' seniority while 79.3% aged under 50 have less than 15 years) but it is age that is eliminated (x^2 Mantel-Haenszel, p = 0.96).

o The redundancy between professor rank and doctoral thesis defended (a professor by definition has already defended a thesis) favoured the thesis, rank was eliminated (X Mantel-Haenszel, p = 0.96). The position of head of department and seniority were also redundant, and the position of head of department was eliminated (%2 Mantel-Haenszel, p = 0.35).

o The variable 'head of department having published an original article as first author' was not introduced into the multivariate analysis model since 35.4% of cases and 17.1% of witnesses were themselves heads of department.

- **A total of 17 variables were introduced (to form the complete model)**
- Table **2** Variables for which **the analysis was continued.**
- Table 3 below shows the results of the final model.

o **Analysis of three-variable tables, each with its own status and two categories (cases and witnesses), revealed an interaction between foreign collaboration and collaboration with a biostatistician and/or epidemiologist (Breslow index test, p = 0.045).**

o **This interaction was introduced into the multivariate analysis model, along with all the variables for which the analysis was carried out.**

was pursued, with the exception of age, professor's grade and head of department.

Model improvement: is calculated from the basic -2 log likelihood *value* (-2LL), which illustrates the difference between the basic model (the constant or event that happens most often) and the model with one or more predictors.

$$\chi^2 = 2[LL\ (\text{modèle}) - LL\ (\text{base})]$$

The difference is squared, because the degree of significance of the result is assessed on the basis of the x distribution^2 (ddl = k-1), where k represents the number of parameters in the model.

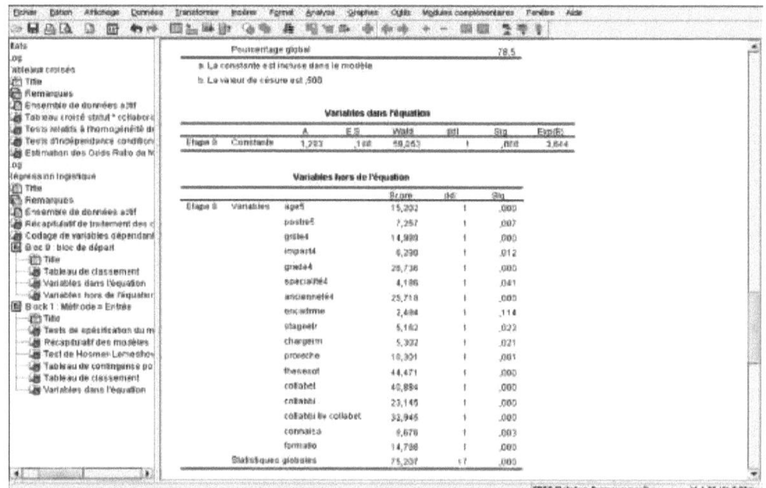

Table 1. Characteristics for which the 49 cases and 193 controls did not differ at the end of the bivariate analysis.

Features	Categories	Case n	Case %	Witnesses n	Witnesses %	OR	95% CI	P
Faculty	Algiers	26	53.1	92	47.7	1.24	0.66-2.33	0.50
	Other	23	46.9	101	52.3	1		
	Total	49	100.0	193	100.0			
Type	Female	24	49.0	88	45.6	1.15	0.61-2.15	0.67
	Male	25	51.0	105	54.4	1		
	Total	49	100.0	193	100.0			
Hospital workload important	No	13	27.1	36	18.9	1.59	0.76-3.31	0.21
	Yes	35	72.9	154	81.1	1		
	Total	48	100.0	190	100.0			
Private sector activity	No	47	95.9	174	91.1	2.30	0.51-10.29	0.42
	Yes	2	4.1	17	8.9	1		
	Total	49		191				
Access to private publishers via Internet	Yes	22	44.9	67	35.3	1.50	0.79-2.82	0.21
	No	27	55.1	123	64.7	1		
	Total	49	100.0	190				
Should a teacher publish in indexed journals	Yes	47	97.9	181	95.8	2.08	0.25-17.02	0.85
	No	1	2.1	8	4.2	1		
	Total	48	100.0	189	100.0			
Does a research project have to be published in an indexed journal?	Yes	46	95.8	182	95.3	1.14	0.24-5.44	1.00
	No	2	4.2	9	4.7	1		
	Total	48	100.0	191	100.0			
Number of teachers in the service (m ± s)	5.98 ±3.94 (n = 48)		6.46 ± 3.23 (n = 191)			Test t (distribution normal)		0.38
Number of assistants in the service (m ± s)	1.94 ± 1.77 (n = 48)		2.60 ±2.68 (n= 190)			Test U de Mann-Whitney		0.26
Number of residents in the service (m ± s)	16.53 ± 16.88 (n=47)		16.12 ± 11.40 (n= 188)			Test U de Mann-Whitney		0.65

Features	Categories	Case		Witnesses		OR	95% CI	p
		n	%	n	%			
Age	> 50 years	29	59.2	63	32.6	2.99	1.57-5.70	$<10^3$
	< 50 years	20	40.8	130	67.4	1		
	Total	49	100.0	193	100.0			
Head of department	Yes	17	34.7	33	17.1	2.58	1.28-5.17	0.007
	No	32	65.3	160	82.9	1		
	Total	49	100.0	193	100.0			
Grade of professor	Yes	24	49.0	28	14.5	5.66	2.84-11.26	$<10^4$
	No	25	51.0	165	85.5	1		
	Total	49	100.0	193	100.0			
Surgeon	No	45	91.8	153	79.3	2.94	1.00-8.66	0.042
	Yes	4	8.2	40	20.7	1		
	Total	49	100.0	193	100.0			
Participation in a research project	Yes	39	81.3	115	60.5	2.83	1.29-6.17	0.007
	No	9	18.7	75	39.5	1		
	Total	48	100.0	190	100.0			
Heavy university load	Yes	39	79.6	117	61.9	2.40	1.13-5.10	0.020
	No	10	20.4	72	38.1	1		
	Total	49	100.0	189	100.0			
Internship abroad (>1 month)	Yes	32	65.3	88	45.8	2.22	1.16-4.27	0.015
	No	17	34.7	104	54.2	1		
	Total	49	100.0	192	100.0			
Supervision of final year dissertations	Yes	46	93.9	162	83.9	2.93	0.86-10.03	0.074
	No	3	6.1	31	16.1	1		
	Total	49	100.0	193	100.0			
Collaboration biostatistician and/or epidemiologist	Yes	36	73.5	64	35.6	5.02	2.48-10.15	$<10^5$
	No	13	26.5	116	64.4	1		
	Total	49	100.0	180	100.0			

Table 3: Bivariate and multivariate analysis of factors ultimately related to teacher output at the end of the analysis

Associated factor	Category	Case		Witnesses		Bi-varied analysis		
		n	%	n	%	OR	95% CI	P
Former as as a teacher	> 15 years	38	77.6	72	37.3	5.81	2.79-12.07	$<10^4$
	< 15 years	11	22.4	121	62.7	1		
The teacher evaluation grid promotes writing	No	34	69.4	63	32.6	4.68	2.37-9.21	$<10^4$
	Yes (and ignore)	15	30.6	130	67.4	1		
These for a doctorate in medical science supported	Yes	41	83.7	60	31.3	11.28	4.98-25.51	$<10^4$
	No	8	16.3	132	68.7	1		
Training in bio-statistics and/or epidemiology	Yes	33	67.3	69	36.5	3.59	1.84-6.99	$<10^3$
	No	16	32.7	120	63.5	1		
Correct knowledge English language	Yes	33	68.8	90	46.6	2.52	1.29-4.93	0.006
	No	15	31.2	103	53.4	1		

Foreign collaboration							
	Yes	32	68.1	35	19.1	9.02	4.41-18.45	<10^5
	No	15	31.9	148	80.9	1		

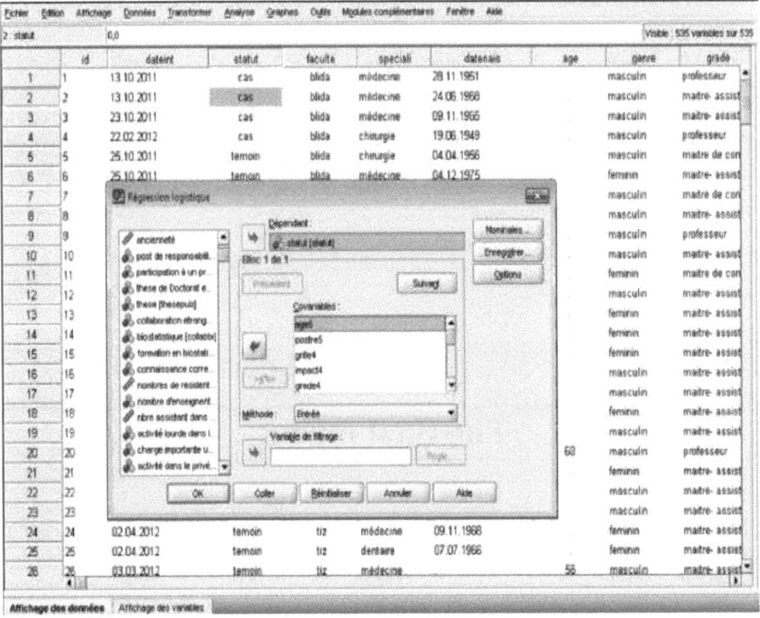

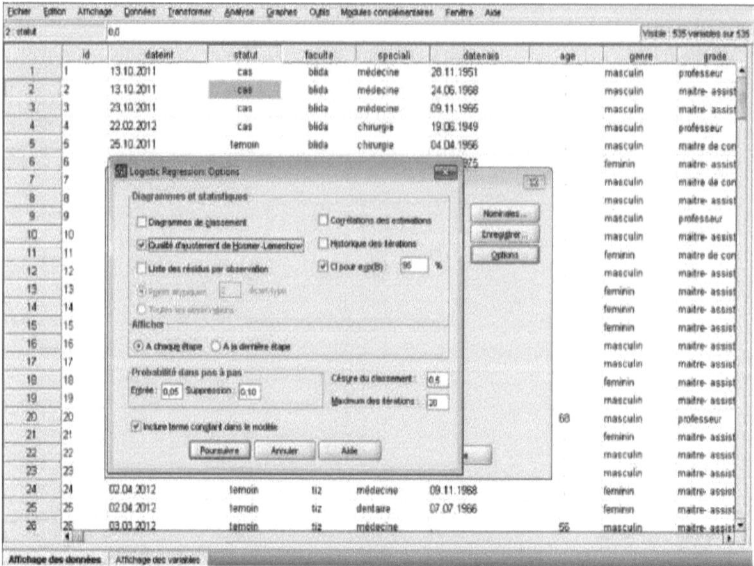

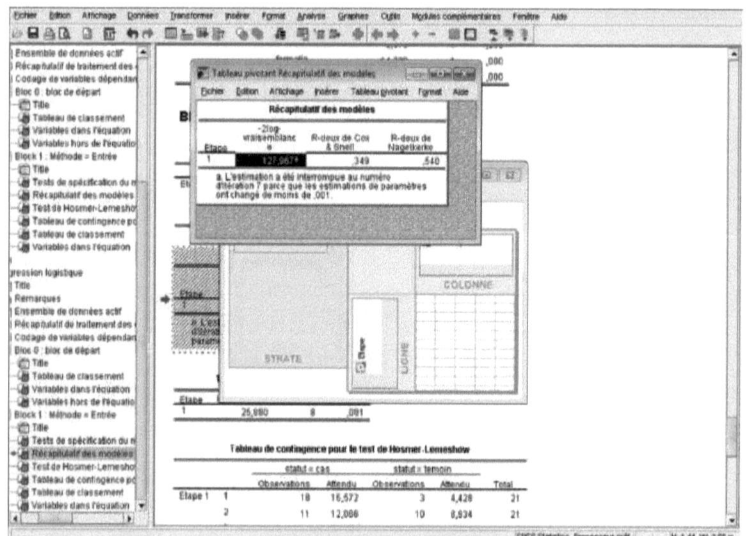

The final model

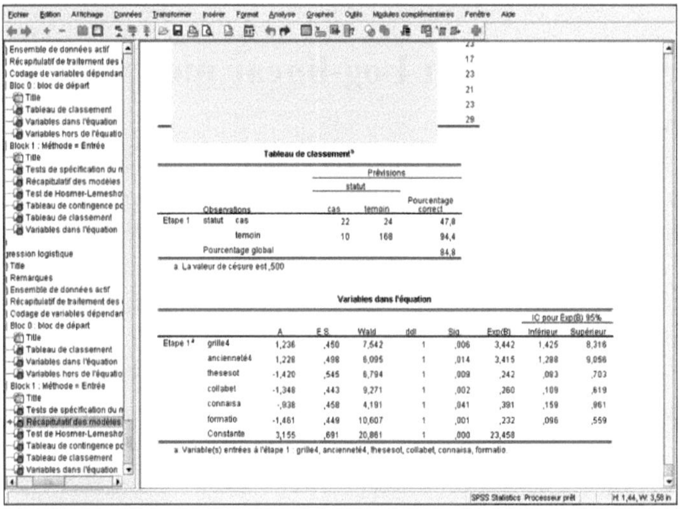

Menu bar: Fichier Édition Affichage Données Transformer Insérer Format Analyse Graphes Outils Modules complémentaires Fenêtre Aide

Navigation pane:
- Ensemble de données actif
- Récapitulatif de traitement des (
- Codage de variables dépendan
- Bloc 0 : bloc de départ
  - Title
  - Tableau de classement
  - Variables dans l'équation
  - Variables hors de l'équatio
- Block 1 : Méthode = Entrée
  - Title
  - Tests de spécification du m
  - Récapitulatif des modèles
  - Test de Hosmer-Lemesho
  - Tableau de contingence po
  - Tableau de classement
  - Variables dans l'équation
- gression logistique
- Title
- Remarques
- Ensemble de données actif
- Récapitulatif de traitement des (
- Codage de variables dépendan
- Bloc 0 : bloc de départ
  - Title
  - Tableau de classement
  - Variables dans l'équation
  - Variables hors de l'équatio
- Block 1 : Méthode = Entrée
  - Title
  - Tests de spécification du m
  - Récapitulatif des modèles
  - Test de Hosmer-Lemesho
  - Tableau de contingence po
  - Tableau de classement
  - Variables dans l'équation

23
17
23
21
23
29

Tableau de classement[a]

| | Observations | | Prévisions | | |
| | | | statut | | Pourcentage correct |
			cas	temoin	
Etape 1	statut	cas	22	24	47,8
		temoin	10	168	94,4
	Pourcentage global				94,8

a. La valeur de césure est ,500

Variables dans l'équation

		A	E.S.	Wald	ddl	Sig.	Exp(B)	IC pour Exp(B) 95% Inférieur	IC pour Exp(B) 95% Supérieur
Etape 1[a]	grille4	1,236	,450	7,542	1	,006	3,442	1,425	8,316
	ancienneté4	1,228	,498	6,095	1	,014	3,415	1,288	9,056
	thesesot	-1,420	,545	6,794	1	,009	,242	,083	,703
	collabet	-1,348	,443	9,271	1	,002	,260	,109	,619
	connaisa	-,938	,458	4,191	1	,041	,391	,159	,961
	formatio	-1,461	,449	10,607	1	,001	,232	,096	,559
	Constante	3,155	,691	20,861	1	,000	23,458		

a. Variable(s) entrées à l'étape 1 : grille4, ancienneté4, thesesot, collabet, connaisa, formatio.

II. Fish regression Log-linear model on SPSS

1. Introduction

Poisson regression belongs to the family of general linear models (GLM), and is one of the multivariate analysis methods alongside logistic regression.

The log-linear model is used to model (understand) the relationship between a response variable consisting of discontinuous quantitative data (count) (dependent or explained variable) and one or more explanatory variables (independent variables).

Assuming that the dependent variable is written as the logarithm of an affine function of the explanatory variables.

$$\text{Log(y)} = \alpha + \text{ß1 X1} + \text{ß2 X2} + \ldots\ldots\ldots + \text{ßn Xn}$$

y: the dependent variable.

X: the explanatory variables.

$\alpha:$ constant.

ß1,ß2,….ßn : B coefficients, which are the logarithms of the relative risks of each explanatory variable X.

Example:

Poisson regression can be used to examine the number of pupils suspended by schools according to predictors such as gender (girls, boys), race (white, black, Asian), mother tongue (Arabic is their first language, Arabic is not their first language) and disability status (disabled, non-disabled).

Here, 'number of suspensions' is the **dependent variable**, while 'gender', 'race', 'language' and 'disability status' are all **independent variables**.

We can therefore write :

$$\text{Log (nbr de suspension)} = \alpha + \text{ß1 genre} + \text{ß2 race} + \text{ß3 langue} + \text{ß4 statut}$$

2. Conditions for using fish regression

1- Our **dependent variable** consists of **count** data: count variables require integer data which must be equal to zero or more (for example, 0, 1, 2, 3, 4, 5, 8, 354, etc.).

Furthermore, it is sometimes suggested that Poisson regression should only be performed when the mean number is a small value (e.g. less than 10). When the number of counts is large, a different type of regression may be more appropriate (e.g. multiple regression).

2- We have **one or more independent variables**, which can be measured on a continuous scale (weight, height....), ordinal (Likert scale, level of education) or nominal / dichotomous and can be roughly classified as categorical variables (gender with two modalities, ethnicity, profession, etc.).

3- You should have **independence of observations**. This means that each observation is independent of the others, i.e. one observation cannot provide any information about another observation. This is a very important assumption. A lack of independent observations is mainly a problem of study design.

One method for testing the possibility of independence of observations is to compare errors based on a standard model with robust errors in order to determine whether there are large differences.

4- The distribution of the dependent variable follows a Poisson distribution. One consequence of this is that the observed and expected counts should be equal (in reality, just very similar). Essentially, this means that the model predicts the observed counts well. This can be tested in a number of ways, but one method is to calculate the expected numbers and plot them against the observed numbers to see if they are similar.

5-The mean and variance of the model are identical. This is a consequence of condition n°4; that there is a Poisson distribution.

For a Poisson distribution, the variance has the same value as the mean. If we meet this condition, we have ***equidispersion***. However, this is often not the case and our data is either over- or under-dispersed.

There are a variety of methods we can use to assess overdispersion. One method is to evaluate the Pearson dispersion statistic. "See the interpretation of table 4 in the results section.

5- he first two conditions can easily be checked. The other conditions (3, 4 and 5) will be checked using SPSS.

3. SPSS test procedure

We are going to illustrate the procedure on SPSS to carry out a Poisson regression assuming that no condition has been violated.

In our example, **"Number of Awards"** is the *dependent variable* which indicates the number of awards obtained by the pupils of a high school in a year, **"Math Score"** is a *continuous predictor variable* and represents the scores of the pupils in their final mathematics exam, **"Programme"** is a *categorical predictor variable* with three levels indicating the type of programme (general, academic and vocational) in which the students were enrolled.

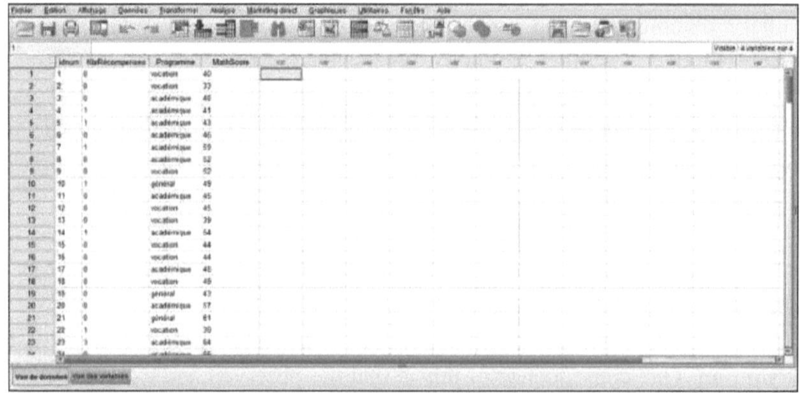

Step 1: Click on **Analysis > General Linear Models > General Linear Models...** in the main menu, as shown below:

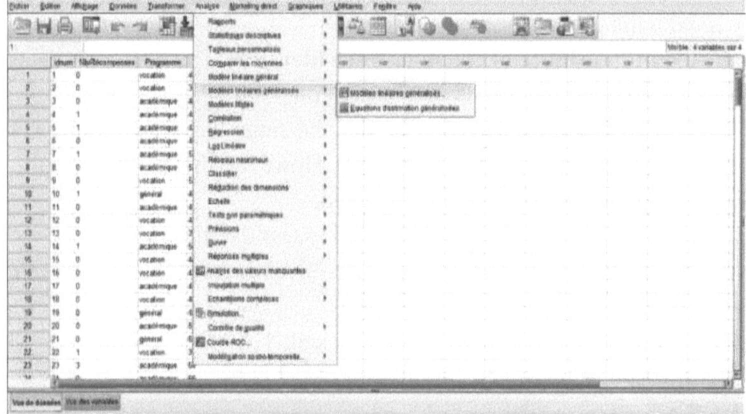

Step 2: After selecting the **"fish log-linear"** model and customising the distribution as a **"fish distribution"** by choosing the **"log"** function, the **General Linear Models** dialog box below will appear:

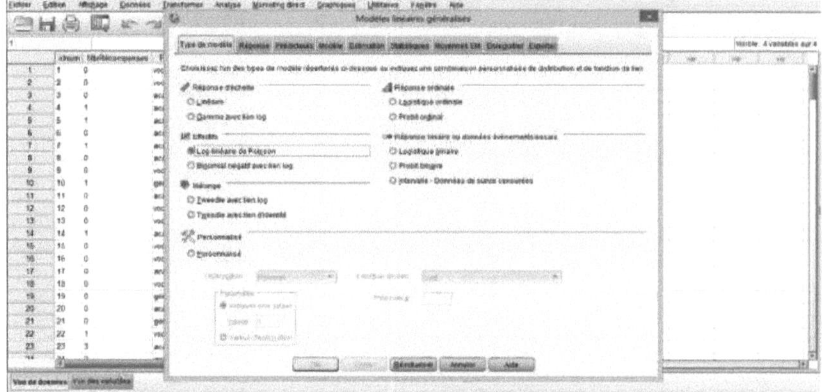

Step 3: Select the **"reply"** tab and you will be presented with the following dialogue box:

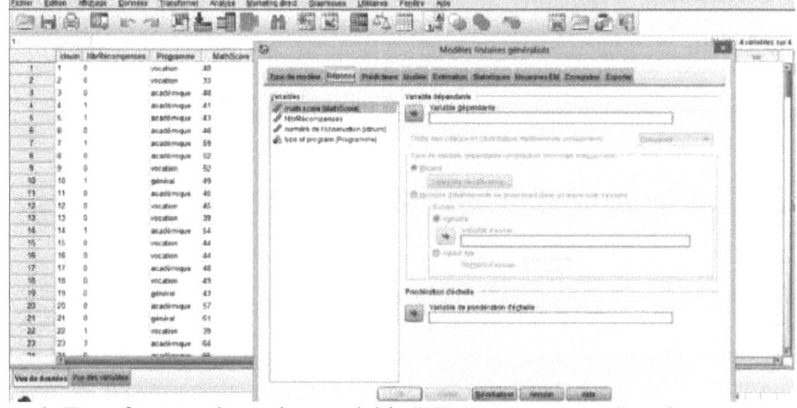

Step 4: Transfer your dependent variable **"NbrRecompenses"** to the "**Dependent variable:**" area using the B button, as shown below:

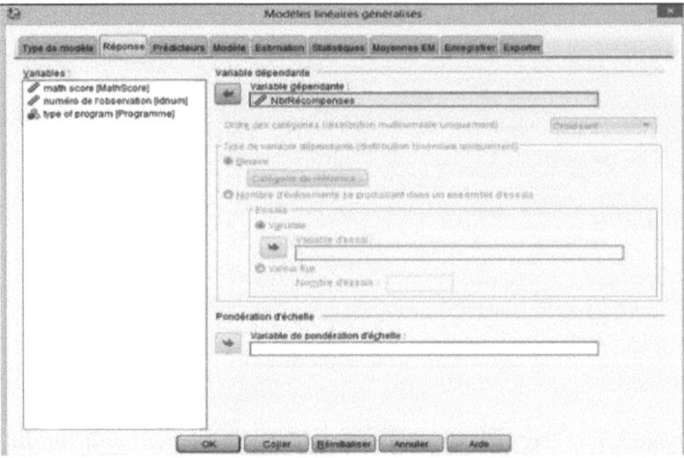

Step 5: Select the **"Predictors"** tab. You will be presented with the following dialog box:

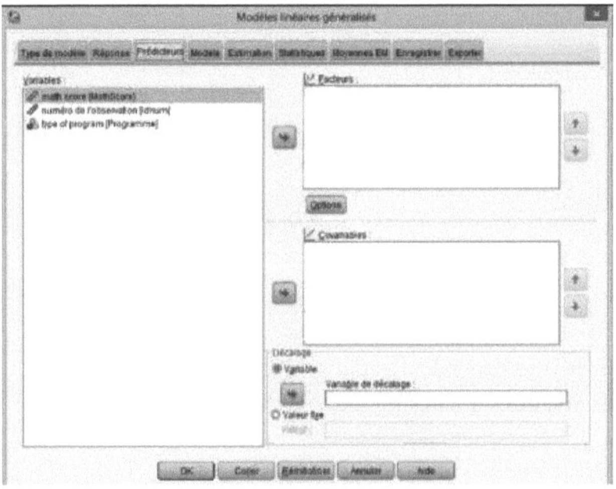

Step 6: Using button B, transfer the categorical independent variable **"programme type"** to the Factors area, and the continuous independent variable, math score, to the Covariates area:

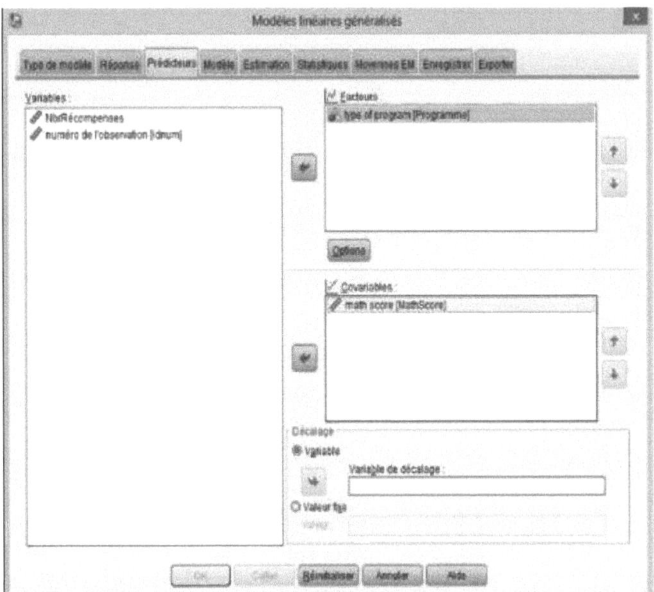

Note: If you have **ordinal** independent variables, you must decide whether they should be treated as categorical and entered in the Factors: box or treated as ordinal independent variables.

Covariates: They cannot be entered in a Poisson regression as ordinal variables.

If you click on the "Options" button, the following dialogue box appears:

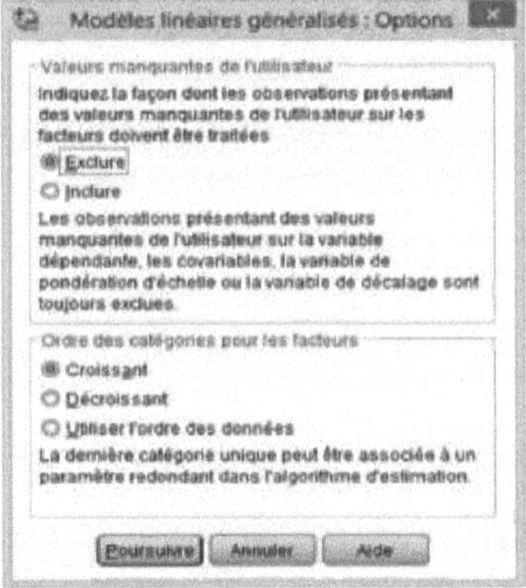

In the **"Order of categories for factors"** area, you can choose between Ascending, Descending and Use data order.

Step 7: Select the **"Model"** tab. Keep the default value for the Main effects region and transfer the independent variables, programme and math score to the **Model:** space using the button as shown below:

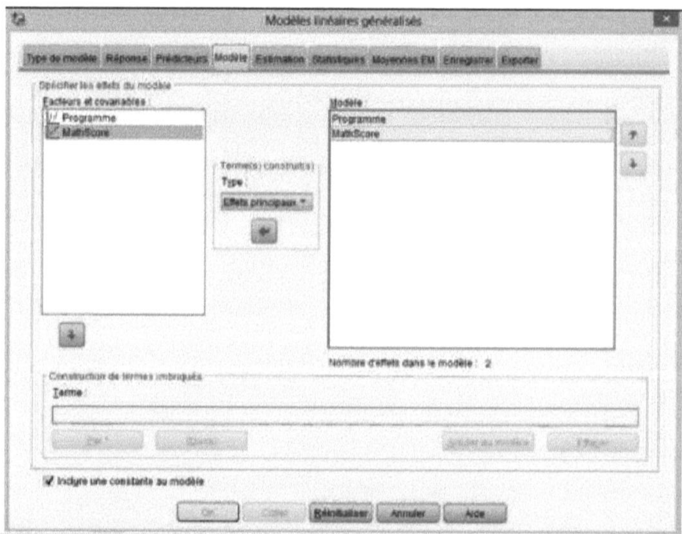

Note: This is where you build your Poisson model. In particular, you determine the **main effect** you have, and if you think you have **interactions** between your independent variables, you include them in your model.

This is important not only to improve the prediction of your model, but also to avoid problems of overdispersion, as outlined in the **"conditions for using fish regression"** section.

Step 8: Select the **"Estimate"** tab and keep the default options, and you will be presented with the dialog box below:

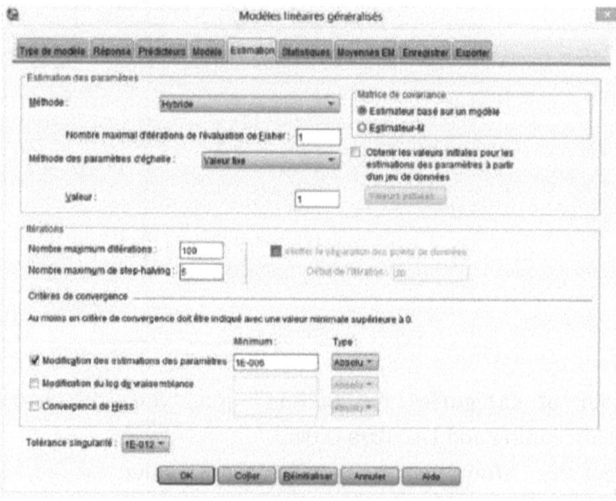

Note: There are a number of different options you can select in the -Estimation- tab, including the ability to choose another option:

• The method of scaling parameters (i.e. **"Deviance"** or **"Pearson's Chi-Square"** instead of "Fixed Value" in the Parameter Estimation space), which could be considered for dealing with overdispersion problems;

• The covariance matrix (i.e. **the -M Robust estimator** instead of the model-based estimator in the Covariance Matrix area), which presents another potential option for dealing with overdispersion problems.

• There are also a number of specifications you can make in the "Iterations" area to deal with non-convergence problems in your Poisson model.

Step 9: Select the **"Statistics"** tab You will be presented with the following dialogue box:

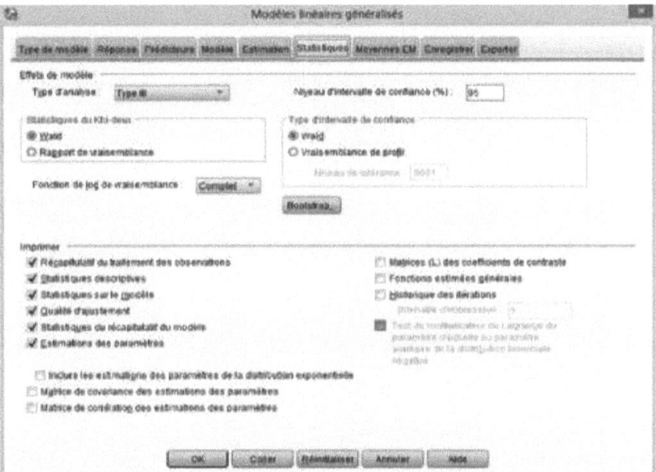

Step 10: Select **"Include estimates of the parameters of the exponential distribution"**.

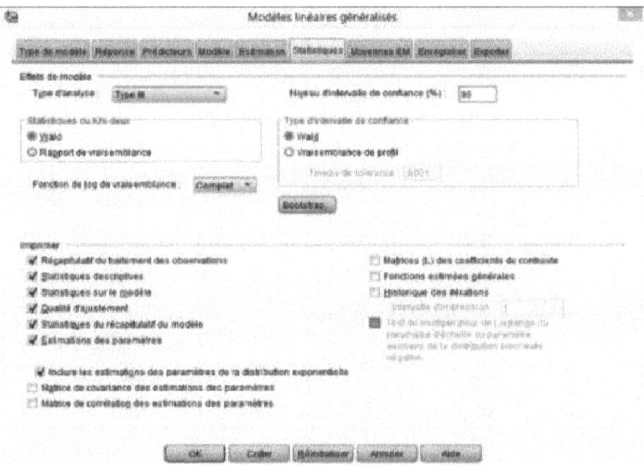

Step 11: You can also select a wide range of other options from the 'EM averages', 'Save' and 'Export' tabs, including important options for examining differences between groups of our categorical variables, as well as for testing the Poisson regression hypotheses.

4. Interpretation of results

We show you the eight tables needed to understand the results of the Poisson regression procedure.

Table 1: Information about the model

Dependent variable	No. of Awards
Probability distribution	Fish
Link function	Log

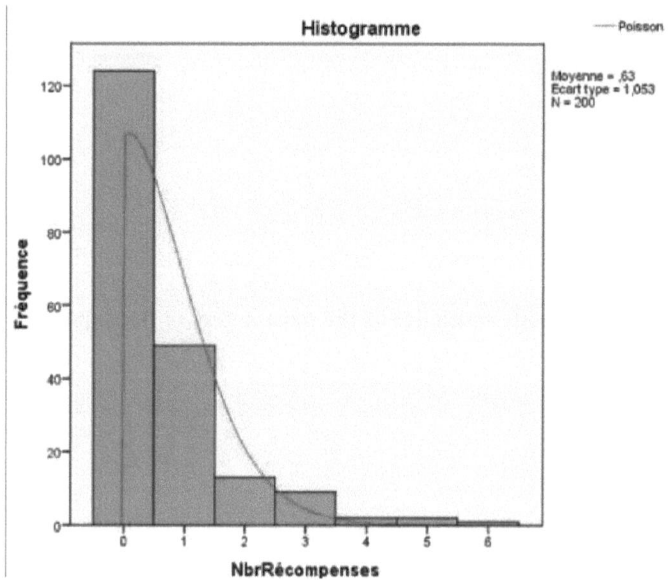

Table 2: Rëcapitulative treatment of observations.

	N	Percentage
Included	200	100,0
Excluded	0	0,0
Total	200	100,0

The second table shows how many observations were included in our analysis (the "Included" row) and how many were not (the "Excluded" row), as well as the percentage of each.

Table 3: Information on the qualitative variable

		N	Percentage
	1- general	45	22,5%
Factor Programme type	2- academic	105	52,5%
	3- vocation	50	25,0%
Total		200	100,0%

The distribution of the modes of the independent variable, which in our example was the 'type of programme', split into three modes (general, academic and vocational).

Table 4: Information on the continuous variable

		N	Minimum	Maximum	Average	Residu type
Dependent variable	Number of awards	200	0	6	,63	1,053
Co-variable	math score	200	33	75	52,64	9,368

- The best we can do from this table is to understand whether there may be over-dispersion in our analysis (verification of *condition 5* of Poisson regression). This can be done by considering the ratio of the variance to the mean of the dependent variable.
- The mean is 0.6 and the variance is 1 (12), giving a ratio of 1 0.6 1.6
- A Poisson distribution assumes a ratio of 1 (i.e. that the mean and variance are equal). Therefore, we can see that before adding explanatory variables, there is a small amount of overdispersion. However, we need to verify this hypothesis when all the independent variables have been added to the Poisson regression.

Determine whether the model corresponds to our data.

Table 5: Quality of fit[a]

	Value	ddl	Value/ddl
Deviance	189,450	196	,967
Deviance scaled up	189,450	196	
Pearson Chi-square	212,144	196	1,082
Pearson Chi-square scaled	212,144	196	
Log likelihood [b]	-182,752		
Akaike Information Criterion (AIC)	373,505		
Small sample corrector (AICC)	373,710		
Bayesian Information Criterion (BIC)	386,698		
AIC coherent (CAIC)	390,698		

Dependent variable : NbrAwards

Model : (Constant), Program, MathScore

a. The information criteria are presented in a smaller, better format.

b. The log likelihood integral function is displayed and is used to calculate the information criteria.

The 'Goodness of Fit' table provides a number of measures that can be used to assess the adequacy of the model and to evaluate the fit of the model. However, we will focus on the value in the **'Value/ ddl'** column for the 'Pearson Chi-square' row, which is '**1.08**', as shown in the table above.

A value of "1" indicates equidispersion, while values greater than "**1**" indicate overdispersion and values less than "**1**" indicate underdispersion. The most common type of violation of the equidispersion condition is overdispersion. With such a small sample size in this example, a value of '1.08' is unlikely to be a serious violation of this assumption.

We evaluate **the deviance (189.45)** as the Chi-square distributed with the degrees of freedom of the model (196). This is not a test of the coefficients of the model, but a test of the shape of the model: Does the shape of the fish model correspond to our data?

We conclude that the model fits reasonably well, because the good quality Chi-square test is not statistically significant (with **196** degrees of freedom, p = **0.204**). If the test had been statistically significant, this would indicate that the data does not fit the model well. In this situation, we can try to determine whether there are any omitted predictor variables, whether our linearity assumption holds and/or whether there is an overdispersion problem.

Table 6: Composite test [a]

Likelihood ratio chi-square	ddl	approx.
98,223	3	,000

Dependent variable : NbrAwards

Model : (Constant), Program, MathScore

a. Compare the adjusted model with the model consisting solely of constants.

The "**Composite Test**": This is a likelihood ratio test to determine whether all the independent variables collectively improve the model relative to **the intercept-only model** (i.e. with no independent variables added or otherwise - all estimated coefficients are zero). With all variables independent in our example model, we have a p-value = 0.000, indicating a statistically significant overall model, as indicated earlier in the "approx" column.

Effects of the model and statistical significance of each independent variable.

You know that adding up all the independent variables generates a statistically significant model, so you will want to know which specific independent variables are statistically significant. Table 7 shows the statistical significance of each of the independent variables in the "approx" column.

Table 7: Model effect tests

Source	Type III		
	Wald chi-square	ddl	approx.
(Constant)	60,442	1	,000

| Programme | 12,306 | 2 | ,002 |
| MathScore | 43,806 | 1 | ,000 |

Dependent variable : NbrRecompenses Model: (Constant), Program, MathScore

- In general, there was no interest in intercepting the model. However, we can see that the 'type of programme' *(p = 0.002)*, and the 'math score' variable *(p = 0.000)*, were statistically significant.
- The 'model effects tests' table evaluates each of the model's variables with the appropriate degrees of freedom.
- The "programme" variable is categorical, with three levels. Thus, they appear in the model as two variables indicating a degree of freedom. To assess the significance of 'programme' as a variable, we need to test these two dummy variables together in a chi-square test at two degrees of freedom. This indicates that 'programme' is a statistically significant predictor *(p = 0.002)* of the dependent variable 'No. of awards'.
- The continuous prediction variable "MathScore" requires a degree of freedom in the model, and the test presented here is equivalent to that in the Parameter Estimates output.

Table 8: Parameter estimates

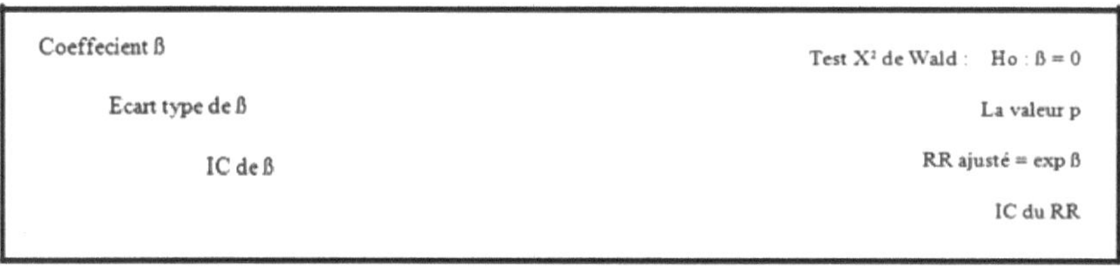

This table provides both the coefficient estimates (the "B" column) of the Poisson regression and the exponential values of the coefficients (the "Exp (B)" column). The latter are generally the most informative. These exponential values can be interpreted in more than one way:
- Consider, for example, the mathematical score obtained (i.e. the "MathScore" range). The exponential of B is **1.073**. This means that the number of rewards (i.e. the number of the dependent variable) will be **1.073 times** greater for each point obtained in mathematics during the year.
- In other words, there is a **7.3% increase in** the number of rewards for each point obtained in mathematics.

The indicator variable [programme = 1] is the expected difference in the number of logs between group 1 and the reference group [programme = 3].

The indicator variable [programme = 2] is the expected difference in the number of logs between group 2 and the reference group.

The expected log count for programme **level 1 decreases** by about **0.37**.

Compared to programme **level 3**, the expected log count for programme **level 2** **increases** by about **0.71**.

5. Fish regression presentation table

	RR ajustes	95% CI		P
		Inf.	Sup.	
Programme 1: general	0.69	0.29	1.64	0.40
Programme 2: academic	2.04	1.09	3.82	0.026
Programme 3: vocation	1		--	
Math Score	1.07	1.05	1.09	0.000

III. Multivariate analysis of variance

1. Definition

ANOVA:

- Dependent variable = 1
- Independent variable > 1

MANOVA :

- Dependent variable > 1
- Independent variable > 1

Association between qualitative variables (independent = x_1, x_2 , x_3 , ...) and quantitative variables (dependent = y_1, y_2 , y_3 ,...)

Dependent variables:

y1 = Survival,

y_2= BMI,

y_3 = The tumour

Independent variables:

x1 = cancer treatment

Why not do 3 ANOVAS? The ***more tests you do, the greater your chances of making a type 1 error.***

MANOVA

- H0: cancer treatment (x_1) is not associated with any of the 3 dependent variables (y_i,y_2,y)$_3$
- Hl: there is an association between x1 and at least one of the variables (y_1,y_2 , y)$_3$

2. SPSS application

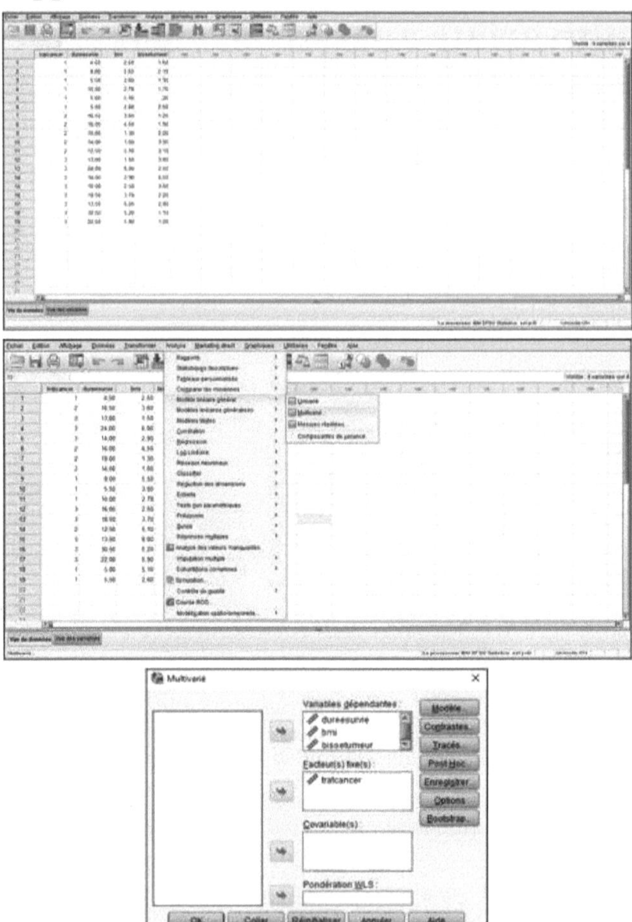

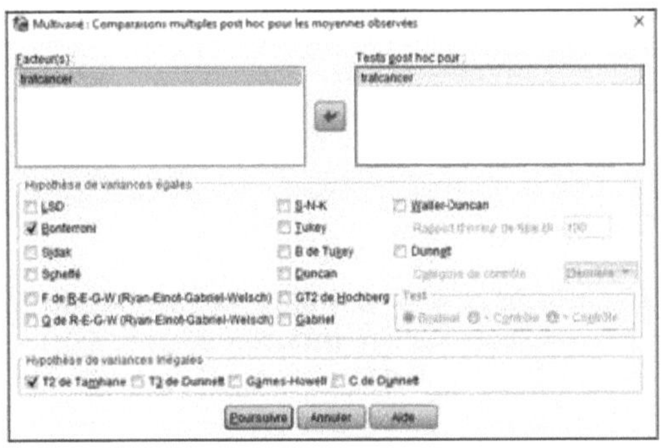

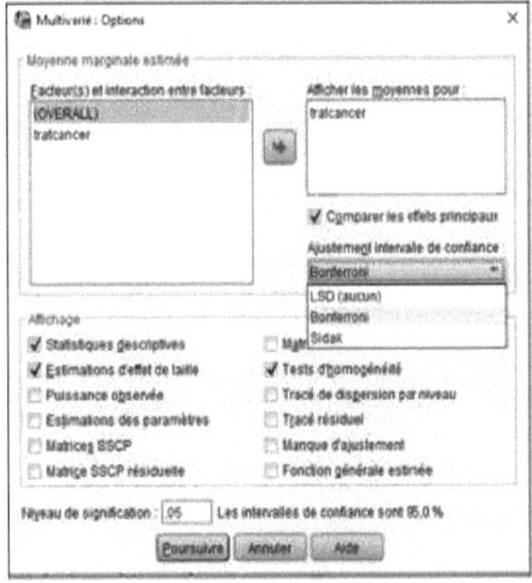

3. SPSS results

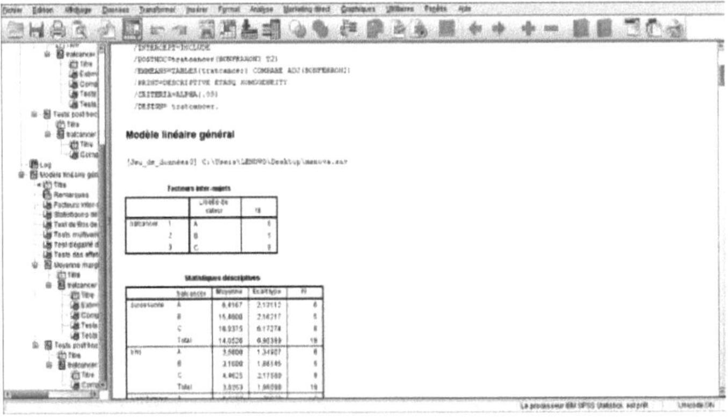

Box test of equality of covariance matrices:

Box test   20,007 1,164 12

F   841,331 **,304**

ddl1

ddl2

Meaning

Tests the null hypothesis that the **observed covariance matrix of** the dependent variables is equal across the **different groups.** a. Design: **Constant + tratcancer**

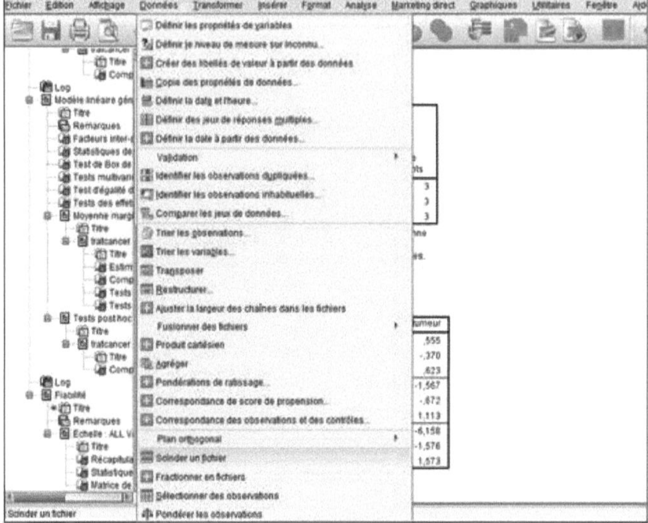

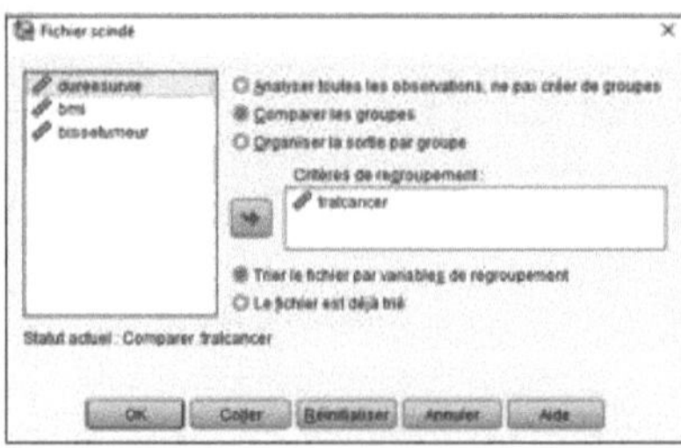

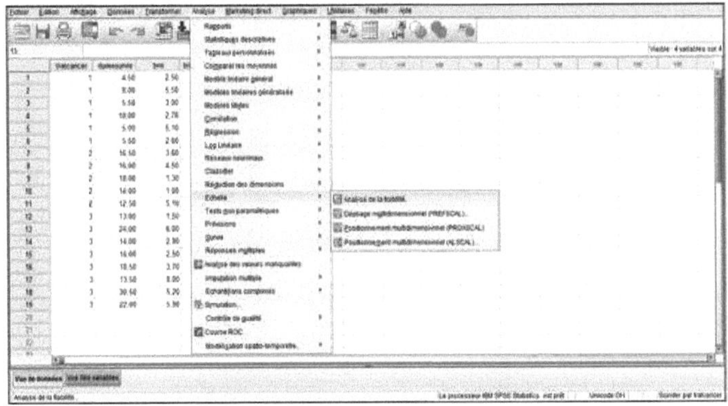

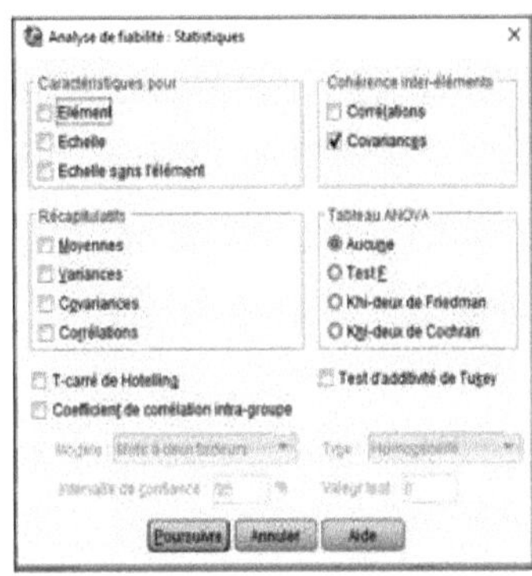

Echelle : ALL VARIABLES

Récapitulatif de traitement des observations

tratcancer			N	%
A	Observations	Valide	6	100,0
		Exclu[a]	0	,0
		Total	6	100,0
B	Observations	Valide	5	100,0
		Exclu[a]	0	,0
		Total	5	100,0
C	Observations	Valide	8	100,0
		Exclu[a]	0	,0
		Total	8	100,0

a. Suppression par liste basée sur toutes les variables de la procédure.

Statistiques de fiabilité

tratcancer	Alpha de Cronbach[a]	Alpha de Cronbach basé sur des éléments standardisés[a]	Nombre d'éléments
A	,184	,084	3
B	-6,674	-23,962	3
C	-,239	-3,221	3

a. La valeur est négative en raison d'une covariance moyenne

Tests multivariés[a]

tratcancer	Effet		Valeur	F	ddl de l'hypothèse	Erreur ddl	Signification	Eta-carré partiel
A	Constante	Trace de Pillai	,959	23,155[b]	3,000	3,000	,014	,959
		Lambda de Wilks	,041	23,155[b]	3,000	3,000	,014	,959
		Trace de Hotelling	23,155	23,155[b]	3,000	3,000	,014	,959
		Plus grande racine de Roy	23,155	23,155[b]	3,000	3,000	,014	,959
	tratcancer	Trace de Pillai	,000	.[b]	,000	,000		
		Lambda de Wilks	1,000	.[b]	,000	4,000		
		Trace de Hotelling	,000	.[b]	,000	2,000		
		Plus grande racine de Roy	,000	,000[b]	3,000	2,000	1,000	,000
B	Constante	Trace de Pillai	,999	957,208[b]	3,000	2,000	,001	,999
		Lambda de Wilks	,001	957,208[b]	3,000	2,000	,001	,999
		Trace de Hotelling	1435,812	957,208[b]	3,000	2,000	,001	,999
		Plus grande racine de Roy	1435,812	957,208[b]	3,000	2,000	,001	,999
	tratcancer	Trace de Pillai	,000	.[b]	,000	,000		
		Lambda de Wilks	1,000	.[b]	,000	3,000		
		Trace de Hotelling	,000	.[b]	,000	2,000		
		Plus grande racine de Roy	,000	,000[b]	3,000	1,000	1,000	,000
C	Constante	Trace de Pillai	,991	193,802[b]	3,000	5,000	,000	,991
		Lambda de Wilks	,009	193,802[b]	3,000	5,000	,000	,991
		Trace de Hotelling	116,281	193,802[b]	3,000	5,000	,000	,991
		Plus grande racine de Roy	116,281	193,802[b]	3,000	5,000	,000	,991
	tratcancer	Trace de Pillai	,000	.[b]	,000	,000		

IV. Quantifying reproducibility

Cohen's kappa, Fleiss' kappa and intra-class correlation coefficients

1. Introduction

The reproducibility of an examination, assessed during a diagnostic reliability study, is its ability to reproduce the same information on a regular basis during repeated measurements, under the same conditions, on the same person.

The more reproducible the test, the more reliable it is.

2. Cohen's Kappa coefficient

In the case of categorical judgements (the judgement criterion is *a qualitative characteristic)*, the rate of agreement or "concordance" is estimated by the Kappa coefficient proposed by Cohen.

This coefficient measures the agreement between **two observers.**

The kappa value can vary from -1 (absolute disagreement) to +1 (total agreement).

The concordance can be assumed to be:

- **Good** if kappa >0.6
- **Bad** if kappa <0.3
- **Intermediate** between these two values.

The following examples are taken from the textbook **"Precis d'epidemiologie, chapitre 17: Reproductibilité des résultats"**.

A. Example 1:

In the example below, we want to measure the reproducibility of a technique for measuring urinary sugar. The results are expressed as negative, weakly positive and positive. The test is performed twice on each patient by two different doctors.

Table 17.2 p 262: Qualitative estimation by two doctors of the presence of sugar in urine in the same group of 70 patients (cross tabulation).

Doctor A Results	Negative	Weakly +	positive	Total
Ndgative	28	14	0	42
Doctor B Weakly +	10	4	6	20
positive	4	2	2	8
Total	42	20	8	70

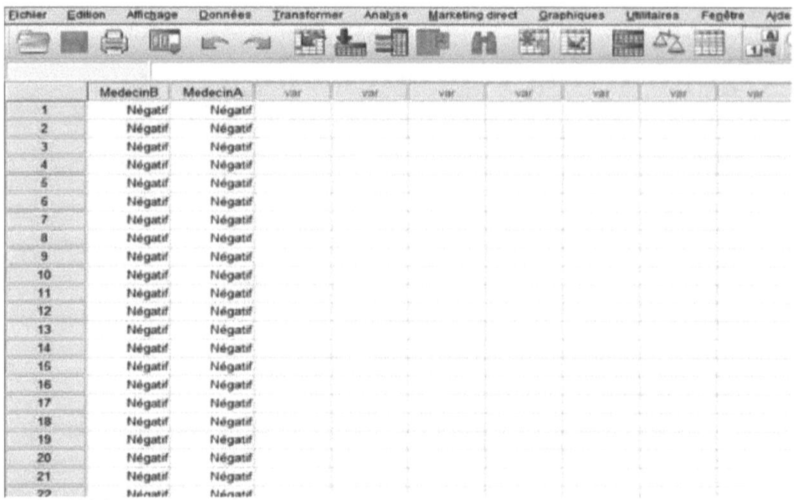

Step 1: Click on **Analysis > Descriptive statistics > Crosstabs** in the main menu, as shown below:

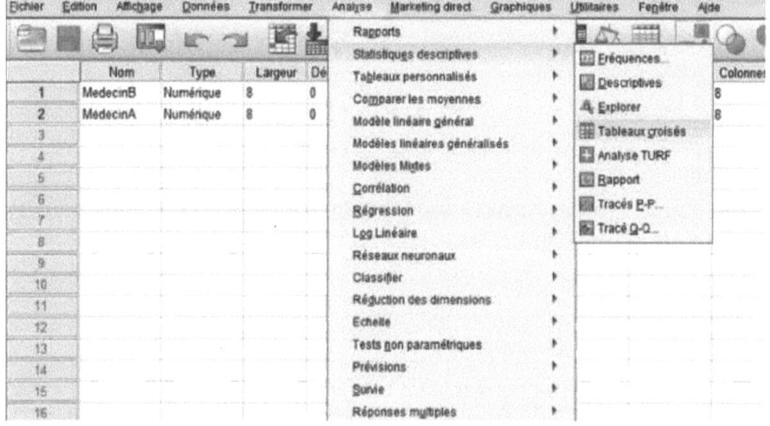

Step 2: After entering the two variables '**results given by doctor B'** and '**results given by doctor A**' in the **'row'** and '**column'** spaces respectively, click on the '**statistics'** button:

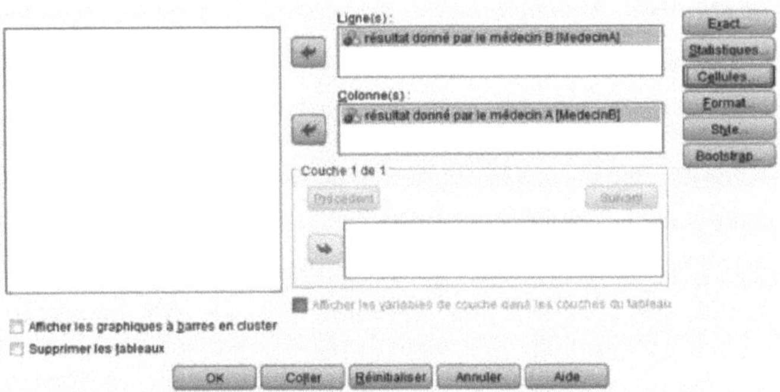

Step 3: Tick the 'kappa' coefficient:

Step 4: Click on **continue** then **ok** to obtain the following results:

Summary of observations

	Comments					
	Valid		Missing		Total	
	N	PdUirCentage	N	Роигс entage	Я	Роиc entage
result given by the doctor B * result given by the IYISd&Cln A	70	100,0%	0	0,0%	70	100,0%

Crosstabulation of results done by the doctor u ' result at tlonne pai le inedecin A

Effect

		results given by doctor A		Total
		Negative	Low - POSitiT	
result given by the doctor B	Ndgative	28	104	42
	Faibiemerrt +	1 4	42	20
	Posilif	0	62	8
Total		42	20S	70

Symmetrical measurements

	Value	Standard asymptotic error[3]	**Approximate Tb**	Approximate **meaning**
Me sure d' accordkappa U Valid comments	.057 70	.093	,612	.540

Meaning of results :

The kappa coefficient in this case was **0.057** (poor agreement between the two doctors).

The null hypothesis consists of saying that there is no agreement between the two doctors (or that the agreement between the two doctors is not significant). In this case the reduced variance given by SPSS (**0.612**) was < 1.96 at the 5% level. Done 1 agreement between the two doctors was non-significant.

We can conclude that there was **poor agreement** between the two doctors. This agreement was non-significant *(p = 0.54)* at the 5% threshold.

B. Example 2:

Two interviewers were asked to classify **126** subjects according to their social class, subdivided into **five classes**. The results are shown in the table below.

Table 17.3 p 264: classification by two interviewers of the same group of 126 subjects according to social class (cross tabulation)

		Interviewer 1					
		CS 1	CS2	CS3	CS4	CS5	Total
	CS 1	18	2	0	2	3	25
	CS2	3	9	0	0	0	12
Interviewer 2	CS3	1	0	11	4	2	18
	CS4	3	1	8	13	1	26
	CS5	2	0	6	11	26	45
	Total	27	12	25	30	32	126

SPSS application :

	Enquêteur2	Enquêteur1	var	var	var	var	var	var	var
1	CS 1	CS 1							
2	CS 1	CS 1							
3	CS 1	CS 1							
4	CS 1	CS 1							
5	CS 1	CS 1							
6	CS 1	CS 1							
7	CS 1	CS 1							
8	CS 1	CS 1							
9	CS 1	CS 1							
10	CS 1	CS 1							
11	CS 1	CS 1							
12	CS 1	CS 1							
13	CS 1	CS 1							
14	CS 1	CS 1							
15	CS 1	CS 1							
16	CS 1	CS 1							
17	CS 1	CS 1							
18	CS 1	CS 1							
19	CS 1	CS 2							
20	CS 1	CS 2							
21	CS 1	CS 4							

Step 1: Click on **Analysis > Descriptive statistics > Cross tabulations** in the main menu, as shown below:

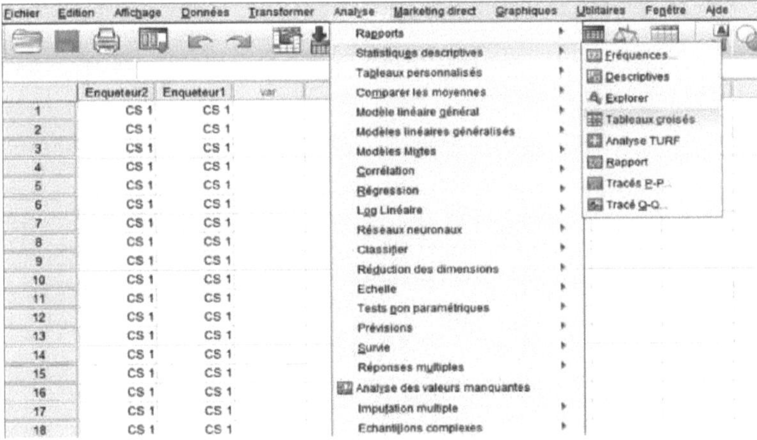

Step 2: After entering the two variables **'CS given by interviewer 2'** and **'CS given by interviewer 1'** in the **'row'** and **'column'** spaces respectively, click on the **'Statistics'** button:

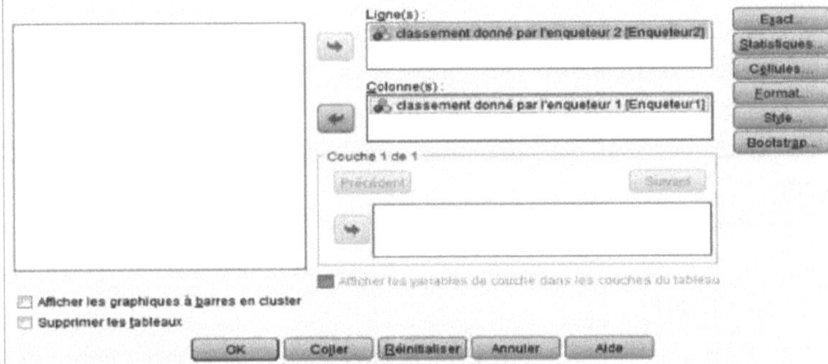

Step 3: Tick the **'kappa'** coefficient

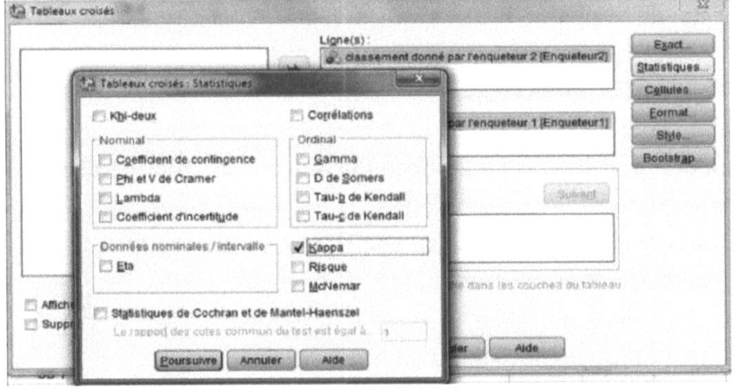

Step 4: Click on **continue** then **ok** to obtain the following results:
Summary of observations

	Comments					
	Valid		Missing		Total	
	N	Percentage	N	Percentage	N	Percentage
ranking given by Surveyor 2 * ranking gives interviewer 1	126	100,0%	0	0,0%	126	100,0%

Cross-tabulated ranking given by interviewer 2 ' ranking given by interviewer 1

Workforce

	classification given by interviewer 1					
	CS 1	CS 2	CS 3	CS 4	CS 5	Total
ranking given by interviewer 2 CS 1	18	2	0	2	3	25
CS 2	3	0	0	0	0	12
CS 3	1	0	11	4	2	18
CS 4	3	1	8	1 3	1	26
CS 5	2	0	6	1 1	26	45
Total	27	12	25	30	32	126

Symmetrical measurements

	Value	Standard asymptotic error [a]	T approximate [b]	Approximate meaning
Measure of agreement Kappa N of valid observations	.502 126	.055	10,919	.000

Meaning of results :

The kappa coefficient in this example was **0.50** (intermediate agreement between the two investigators).

The null hypothesis consists of saying that there is no agreement between the two interviewers (or that the agreement between the two interviewers is not significant).

In this case, the reduced variance given by SPSS (**10.92**) was > 1.96 at the 5% threshold. The agreement between the two investigators was therefore highly significant (**p < 0.001**).

We can conclude that there is an **intermediate level of agreement** between the two investigators.

This agreement was highly significant (**p < 0.001**) at the 5% threshold.

3. Fleiss kappa coefficient

Fleiss' Kappa coefficient is a statistical measure that evaluates agreement for a certain number of observers (> 2) when the judgement criterion being studied is qualitative.

This contrasts with Cohen's kappa coefficient, which only works to assess agreement between two observers.

This coefficient does not exist in the 23[eme] version of SPSS, so you need to download it by following the steps below:

(**Utilities > Extension bundles > Download and install extension bundles... > search for 'kappa de Fleiss' in the search box > Download**).

The Fleiss kappa will be installed systematically on SPSS.

- . Example :

Table **17.4 on p 266** gives the marks (out of 20) given by three examiners to 47 epidemiology examination papers and the qualitative assessment (complete, partially complete, incomplete) given by the three examiners to the single graph in the examination.

To judge the reproducibility of the assessment of the graph by the three examiners A, B and C, a Fleiss kappa must be determined.

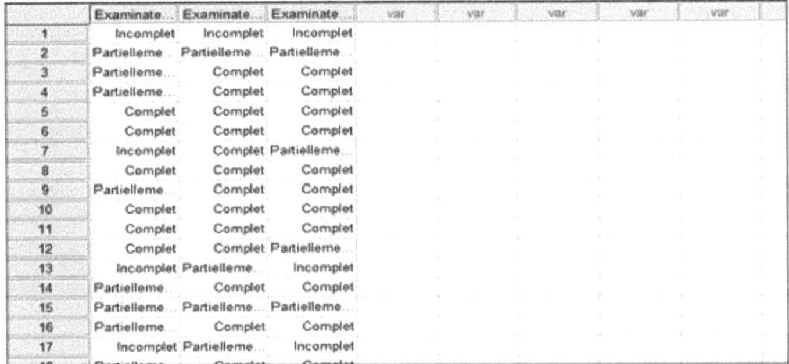

Step 1: Click on **Analyse > Echelle > Fleiss kappa** in the main menu, as shown below:

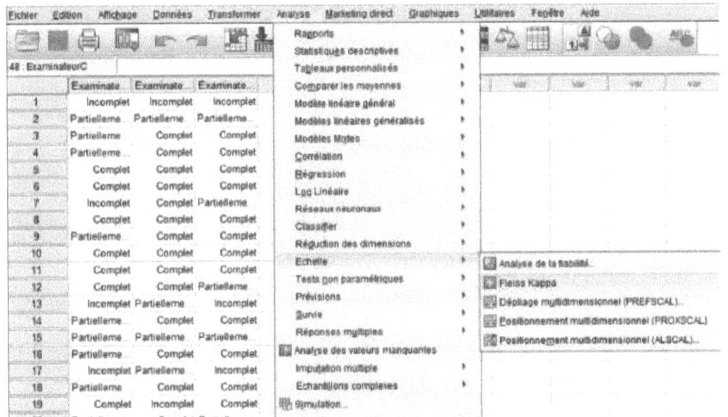

Step 2: After entering the three variables **'rating by A', 'rating by B'** and **'rating by C' in the 'Rating variables'** space, click on **'OK'**:

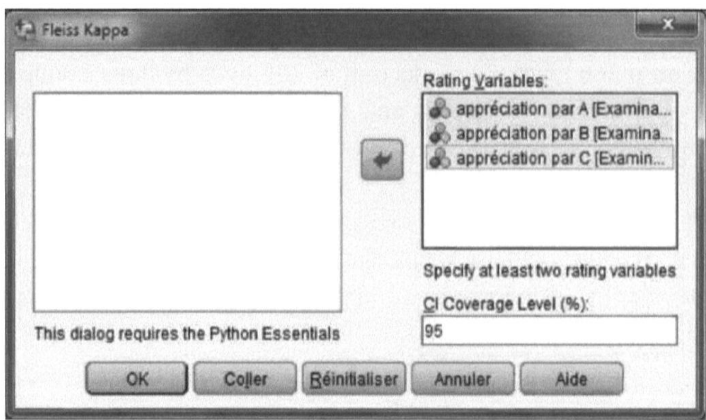

Step 3: Click on **OK** to get the following results:

Overall Kappa

	Kappa	Asymptotic Standard Error	Z	P Value	Lower 95% Asymptotic CI Bound	Upper 95% Asymptotic CI Bound
Overall	.305	.061	4,967	,000	,185	.425

Kappas for **Individual** Categories

Rating Category	Conditional Probability	Kappa	Asymptotic Standard Error	Z	P Value	Lower 95% Asymptotic CI Bound	Upper 95% Asymptotic CI Bound
1	.684	,315	.084	3,740	,000	.150	,480
2	,333	,105	.084	1,244	.214	-.060	,270
3	,621	.522	,084	6,204	,000	,357	,688

Meaning of results :
* Fleiss kappa (for the three categories) = 0.305 (0.185 - 0.425)
* Agreement between the three examiners was significant (Z = 4.97; *p* <0.001).

4. intra-class correlation coefficient

The intra-class correlation coefficient is used to quantify the agreement between 2 or more observers when the measurement is expressed on a quantitative variable.

This coefficient varies between **0** 'agreement due to chance' and **1** 'total agreement between observers'.

A. Example:

The previous example (the one in table **17.4 p 266**) contains data relating to the marks (out of 20) that the three examiners A, B and C gave to 47 epidemiology examination papers.

As the examination mark is quantitative, the intra-class correlation coefficient must be determined to quantify the agreement between the three examiners 'A', 'B' and 'C'.

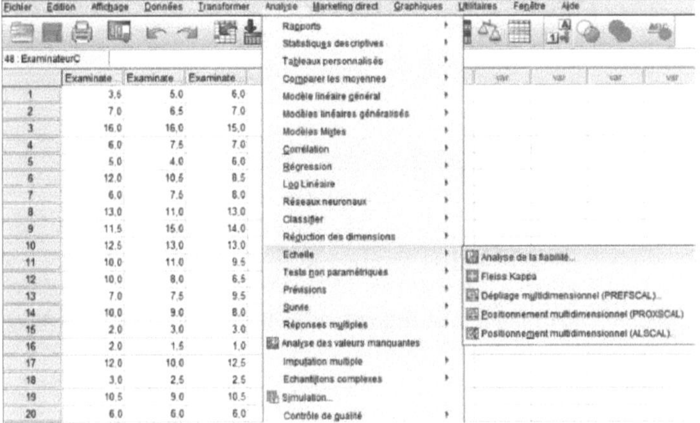

Step 1: Click on **Analyse > Scale > Reliability analysis** in the menu as shown below:

Step 2: After entering the three variables **'appreciation by A'**, **'appreciation by B'** and **'appreciation by C'** in the **'Elements'** space, click on **Statistics**:

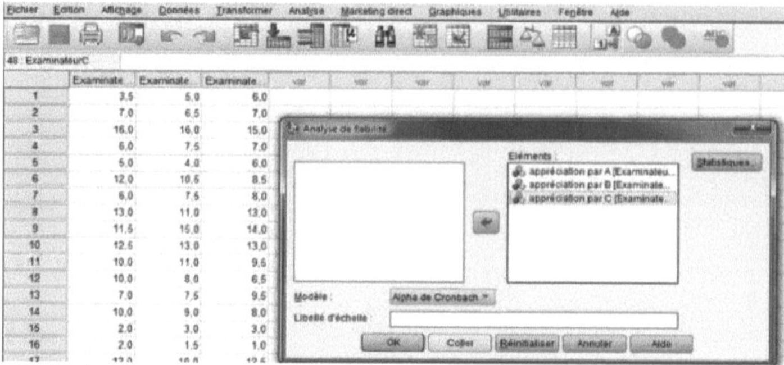

Step 3: Tick the '**intra-group correlation coefficient' box** and click on '**continue**' then '**OK**' to get the results:

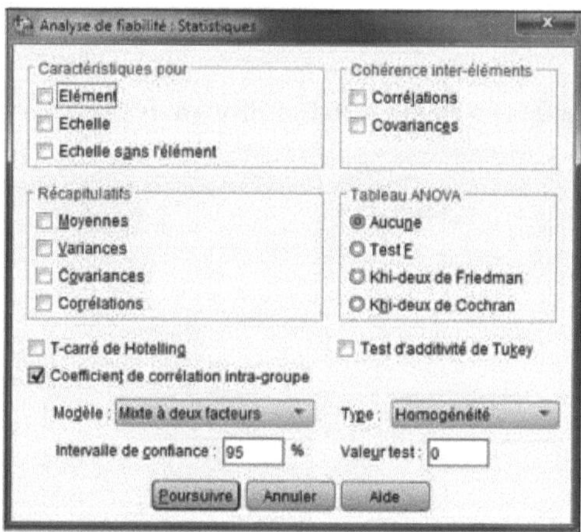

Step 4: Click on OK to obtain the following results:

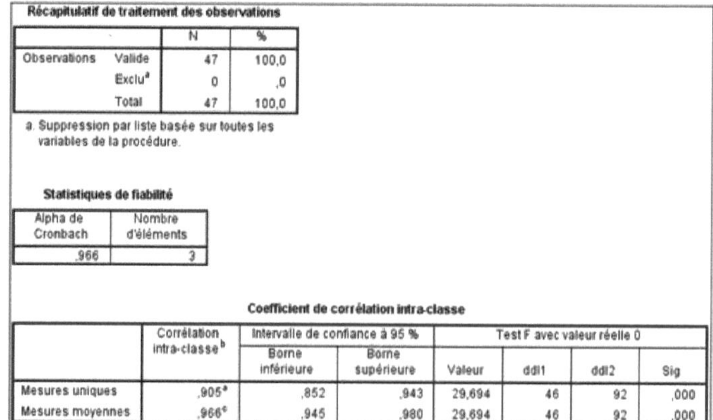

Récapitulatif de traitement des observations

		N	%
Observations	Valide	47	100,0
	Exclu[a]	0	,0
	Total	47	100,0

a. Suppression par liste basée sur toutes les variables de la procédure.

Statistiques de fiabilité

Alpha de Cronbach	Nombre d'éléments
,966	3

Coefficient de corrélation intra-classe

	Corrélation intra-classe[b]	Intervalle de confiance à 95 %		Test F avec valeur réelle 0			
		Borne inférieure	Borne supérieure	Valeur	ddl1	ddl2	Sig
Mesures uniques	,905[a]	,852	,943	29,694	46	92	,000
Mesures moyennes	,966[c]	,945	,980	29,694	46	92	,000

Meaning of results :

Tableau 1 : (descriptive statistics)

- We first obtain a table specifying the number of observations included in the analysis. In our example, we see that 100% of the 47 observations were retained. This means that there were no missing values in the database.

Tableau 2 Cronbach's alpha

• It contains the value of Cronbach's alpha index. We note here that the value of the coefficient is **0.966**, which is excellent, since it exceeds the minimum required threshold of **0.70** (Nunnaly, 1978). This marker is arbitrary, but widely accepted by the scientific community.

• As a result, we can say that, for this scale made up of three observers, we obtain satisfactory internal consistency.

Tableau 3 (intra-class correlation coefficient)

- The intra-class correlation coefficient was **0.905 (0.852 - 0.943)**.

The agreement between the three examiners was very good and the hypothesis that there was no agreement between the three examiners was rejected *(p <* **0.001**).

V. Survival analysis

Survival is a problem that is studied extensively when it comes to **describing the evolution of groups** of sick subjects.

The survival criterion is also often used to compare two groups of patients, as may be the case in therapeutic trials.

The various techniques described, although called survival methods, apply to any event occurring over time (recurrence of a disease, appearance of metastases, complications, sequelae, infections, etc.), and not only, as in the case of survival, to the occurrence of a death.

The corresponding estimated rates are recurrence-free, metastasis-free, complication-free and sequelae-free rates for the successive timeframes used.

Survival time analysis: these methods make it possible to study the time taken for an event to occur if its occurrence is not constant.

• Delay in the eventual occurrence of the death event; but also study all the so-called right-censored data (i.e. the appearance over time of an event with "incomplete" observations made by subjects in whom the event has not yet occurred at the time of analysis.

• The aim of a study may be to find out whether a disease will lead to death or not, but more frequently, we also want to know when this eventual death will occur.

1. Principle of survival analysis

Survival analyses **always** study two variables together:

• A qualitative variable is **"always" binary**.

• A quantitative variable that is **"always" Time.**

2. Definitions

A. Censorship on the left:

At time "t", the event has already occurred (before event t).

B. Censorship on the right:

At time "t" the event has not occurred (after event t)

C. Competing event:

Die of a disease not included in the study

3. The information needed to draw up a survival curve

• The date of origin: this is the date on which the patient entered the study, from which monitoring began.

• The date of last news, which is the most recent date on which we were able to have news of the subject with regard to the criterion under study (dead/alive

....). This date corresponds to the date of the last consultation for subjects who are still alive, or to the date of death for subjects who are deceased.

• Based on the date of the last news item, the date of origin and the status of the subject in terms of the criterion being studied, it is possible to define :

■ Hindsight: this is the period of time between the original date and the point date.

■ Participation time: this is the time corresponding to the entire duration of the monitoring and will be used to establish the survival curve.

• If the last news date is prior to the point date, this date will be used to calculate the participation time.

• If the last news date is after the point date, this date will be used to calculate the participation time.

• If the subject has died at the point date, the participation time measures his or her exact survival.

• If the subject is alive, this period is less than its survival time, in which case the data is said to be right-censored.

• Right-censored" data can correspond to two types of subject:

■ those lost to view who escape the regular surveillance to which they should be subject,

■ Excluded living subjects who are regularly monitored and alive at the point date.

4. Survival analysis

Several methods are used, and we will look at just one non-parametric method: the Kaplan-Meier method.

A. Estimation of survival rate :

• Survival rates are estimated by calculating conditional probabilities.

• These conditional probabilities are simply estimated as the ratio of the number of subjects alive at the end of day D (end of interval) to the number of subjects alive (exposed to the risk of death) at the start of that same day (start of interval).

P (A / B) = P (A Ç B)/ P(b) P(B) # 0

• Estimate of survival, taking into account the different participation times ending with the 3 events listed above.

• On days when no death occurs, the corresponding conditional probability estimates are equal to 1.

• We are therefore only interested in the days on which deaths occur.

• Time is thus divided into unequal intervals beginning at the moment of one death and ending just before the next.

B. The survival function :

Survival rates are calculated as follows:

S(t): estimate of the probability of being alive.

- Being alive until "D" day means surviving on "D" day knowing that you were alive on "D-1" day.

More generally, to be alive until time ti [S (ti)] is:

$$S(t) = S_1 * S_{2/1} * S_{3/2} * \ldots * S_{ti/ti-1}$$

$$S_{(ti/ti-1)} = 1 - \frac{D_i}{N_i} = \frac{N_i - D_i}{N_i}$$

- Ni= number of people at risk of dying at time ti
- Di= number of deaths observed at time ti
- S(t)= S1XS2/1XS3/2 Sti/ti-i
- S(t) is the cumulative probability of survival

C. Survival curve :

The probability of surviving beyond **Ti is** written as P (survive beyond Ti) = P (survive beyond Ti / survive to at least Ti-1).

- P(survival beyond Ti-1)
- Si = Si-1.

D. Median survival time:

- The time "t" for which the probability of survival S(t) is equal to 0.5 (St = 0.5).
- The median time may not be very accurate when it is framed by two **"distant"** events.
- Survival rates will be accompanied by their confidence interval, usually at 95%.
- Variance de Greenwood s'ecrit:

$$var(S)_t = S^2_{(t)} \left[\frac{D_1}{(N_1 - D_1) * N_1} \right] + \ldots + \left[\frac{D_i}{(N_i - D_i) * N_i} \right]$$

E. The Log Rank Test $^{: \approx \chi2 \; à \; k\text{-}1 \; ddl}$

This test applies when the 2 survival curves are calculated using the Kaplan-Meier method.

- H_0 = the two survival curves have identical profiles, so the risk of "death" at a given time is the same in both groups.
- H_1 = the two survival curves have different profiles

A theoretical probability of "death" at time i is calculated:

for example.

$$P_i = (D_{1i} + D_{2i}) / (V_{1i} + V_{2i})$$

This is used to calculate the number of "deaths" in each group at time i:

$$c1i = P_i * V_{1i} \qquad c_{2i} = P_i * V_{2i}$$

We note $c_1 = \Sigma c_{1i}, c_2 = \Sigma c_{2i}, o_1 = \Sigma D_1$ et $o_2 = \Sigma D_2$

5. SPSS application

To carry out a survival analysis, click on Analysis, Survival, Kaplan-Meier,
In the first time dialog box, enter the delay or time for
participation, insert the variable status is defined the event (alive, deceased or remission, relapse etc)
Choose Critere to compare survival between two treatments, for example,
Choose Strate to determine survival under a single treatment with
The button Compares the factors between two by using a test (test log
Rank , Breslow and others).

The Enregistrer... button to determine survival, cumulative frequency.

The Options button to determine the survival table, mean and median survival, diagram (survival and others)

Then click on the Poursuivre

At the end click on the button OK

The different SPSS stages

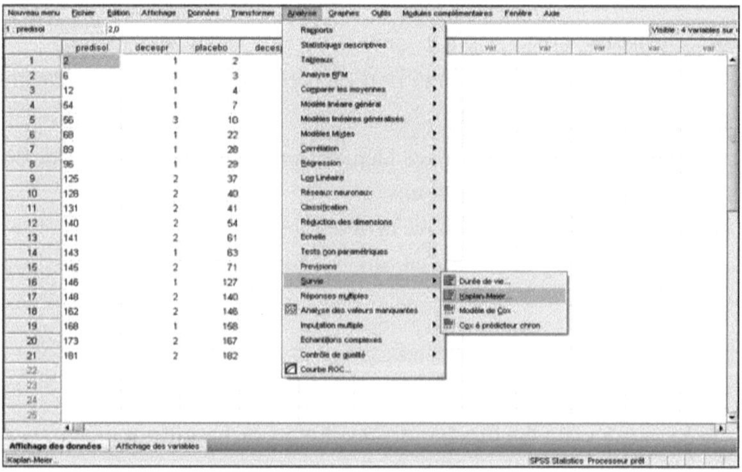

Nouveau menu   Fichier   Édition   Affichage   Données   Transformer   Analyse   Graphes   Outils   Modules complémentaires   Fenêtre   Aide
1 : predisol   2,0
Visible : 4 variables sur
predisol   decespr   placebo   deces   var   var   var   var   var
1   2   1   2
2   6   1   3
3   12   1   4
4   54   1   7
5   56   3   10
6   68   1   22
7   89   1   28
8   96   1   29
9   125 2   37
10   128 2   40
11   131 2   41
12   140 2   54
13   141 2   61
14   143 1   63
15   145 2   71
16   146 1   127
17   148 2   140
18   162 2   146
19   168 1   168
20   173 2   167
21   181 2   182
22
23
24
25

Rapports
Statistiques descriptives
Tableaux
Analyse RFM
Comparer les moyennes
Modèle linéaire général
Modèles linéaires généralisés
Modèles Mixtes
Corrélation
Régression
Log Linéaire
Réseaux neuronaux
Classification
Réduction des dimensions
Echelle
Tests non paramétriques
Prévisions
Survie
Réponses multiples
Analyse des valeurs manquantes
Imputation multiple
Echantillons complexes
Contrôle de qualité
Courbe ROC...

Durée de vie...
Kaplan-Meier
Modèle de Cox
Cox à prédicteur chron

Affichage des données   Affichage des variables
Kaplan-Meier
SPSS Statistics Processeur prêt

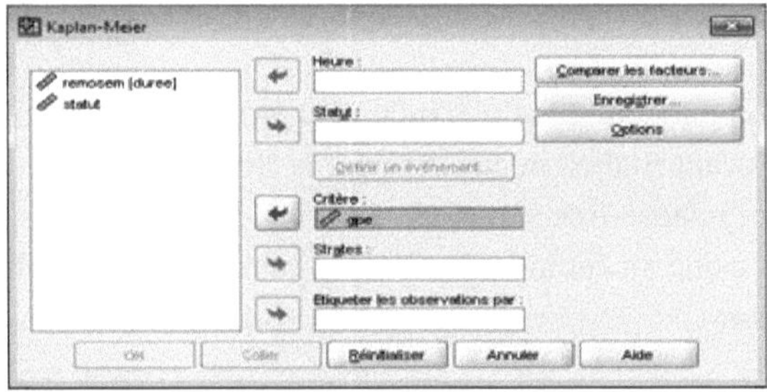

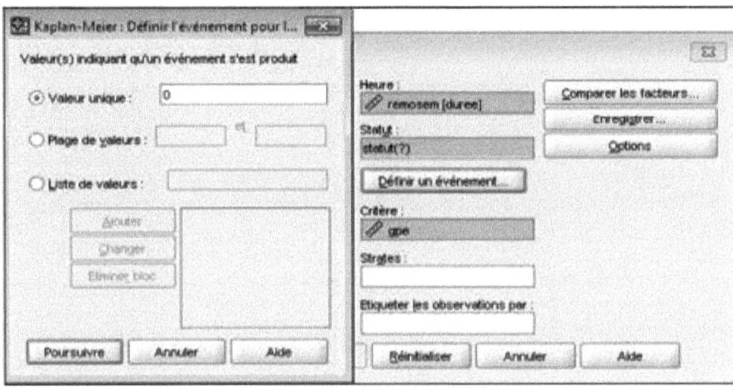

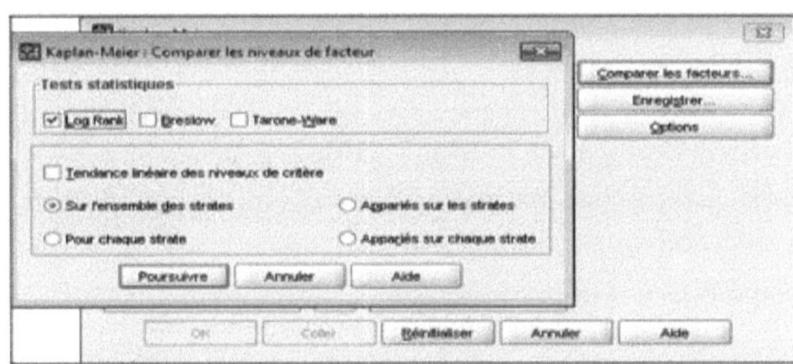

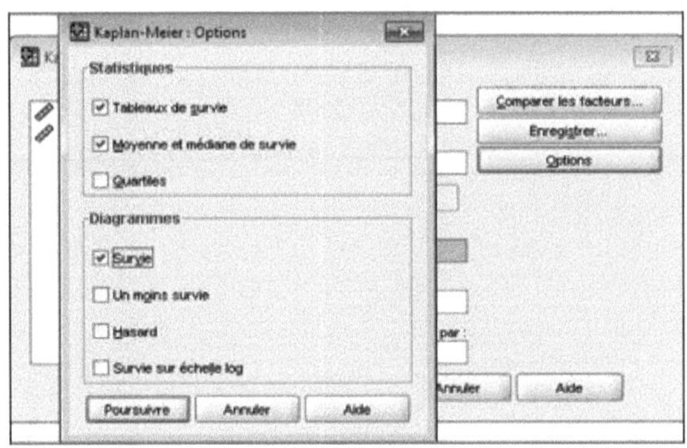

A. Example 1:

- Graphical comparison of the two treatment groups (placebo and trt 6MP; we assume that the event studied in our example is "Relapse";
- Estimation of relapse-free survival ;
- Comparison using an appropriate test (log-rank test) (see application below);

SPSS application:

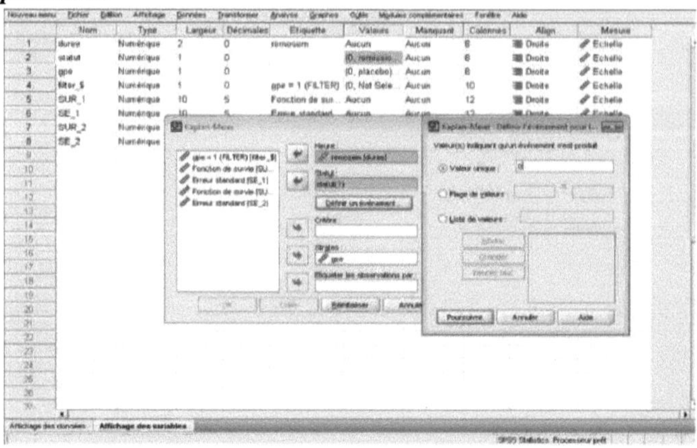

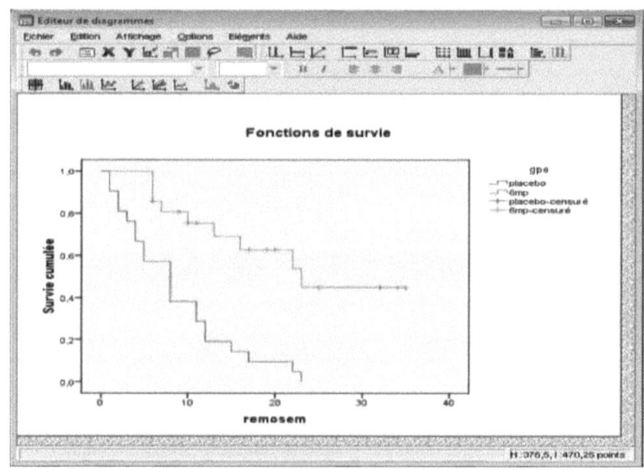

Results

Fonctions de survie
gpe
placebo
6mp
placebo-censuré
6mp-censuré
Survie cumulée
remosem

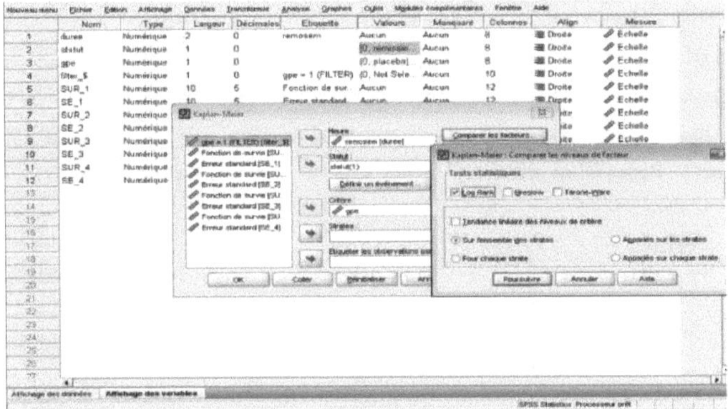

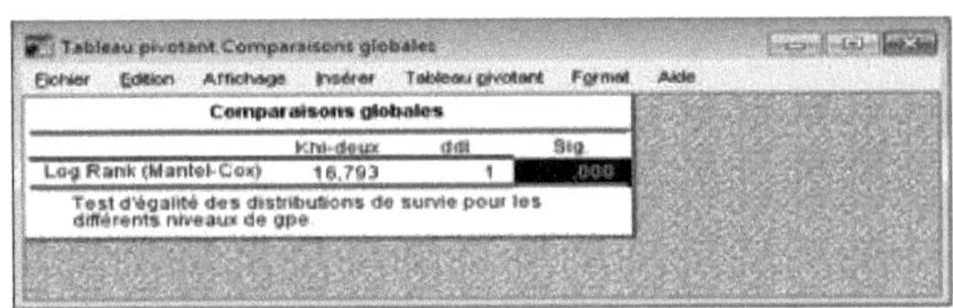

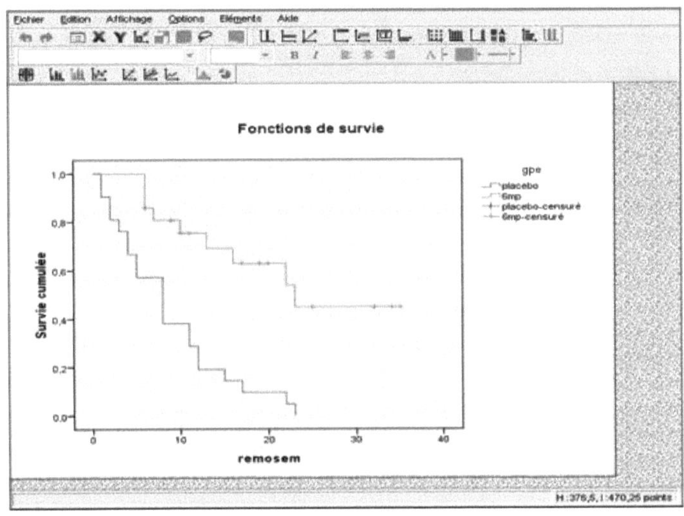

B. Example 2:

At the end of a therapeutic trial in which 5 subjects received treatment A and 5 other subjects treatment B, the following results were obtained:

Table : Results of a randomised therapeutic trial comparing two treatments

Subject no.	Processing allocates	Result	
		Participation time	Status
1	A	14 weeks	ddcddd
2	B	12 weeks	ddcddd
3	B	18 weeks	ddcddd
4	A	9 weeks	ddcddd
5	A	9 weeks	decode
6	A	18 weeks	deceased
7	B	24 weeks	still alive
8	B	20 weeks	still alive
9	A	17 weeks	still alive
10	B	12 weeks	deceased

Using the Kaplan Meier method, we will construct the simplified survival table and the survival curve for :

- The group of patients treated by A,
- The group of patients treated by B.

Next, we will make an overall comparison of the two survival curves.

Simplified survival table for group A

Interval number	Interval	Number of subjects at risk	Number of deaths in the interval	Probability of conditional survival	Cumulative probability of survival
1	[0- 9[	5	0	1	1
2	[9 - 14 [	5	2	0.6000	0.6000
3	[14- 18 [	3	1	0.6667	0.4000
4	18	1	1	0	0

Simplified survival table for group B

Interval number	Interval	Number of subjects at risk	Number of deaths in the interval	Probability of conditional survival	Cumulative probability of survival
1	[0-12[	5	0	1	1
2	[12-18[	5	2	0.6000	0.6000
3	[18-24[	3	1	0.6666	0.4000

Overall comparison of the two survival curves

Time interval between deaths	Deaths in group A O_{Ai}	Deaths in group B O_{Bi}	Subjects featured in A A_i	Subjects featured in B n_{Bi}	Expected number of deaths in A	Expected number of deaths in B

					(E_A)	(E_Bi)
9- 10	2	0	5	5	1	1
12- 13	0	2	3	5	0.75	1.25
14- 15	1	0	3	3	0.5	0.5
18 - 19	1	1	1	3	0.5	1.5
Total	O_A	O_B			E_A = **2.75**	E_B =**4.25**

The Logrank test allows an overall comparison of the two survival curves:

$$\chi^2 = (O_A - E_A)^2 / E_A + (O_B - E_B)^2 / E_B$$

$$\chi^2 = (4\text{-}2.75)^2/2.75 + (3\text{-}4.25)^2/4.25 = 0.5682 + .3676 = 0.94 ; NS$$

The two treatments did not differ significantly.

The two curves do not intersect (*see SPSS application below*), so it was legitimate to run a global test to compare them.

SPSS application:

Presentation of variables :

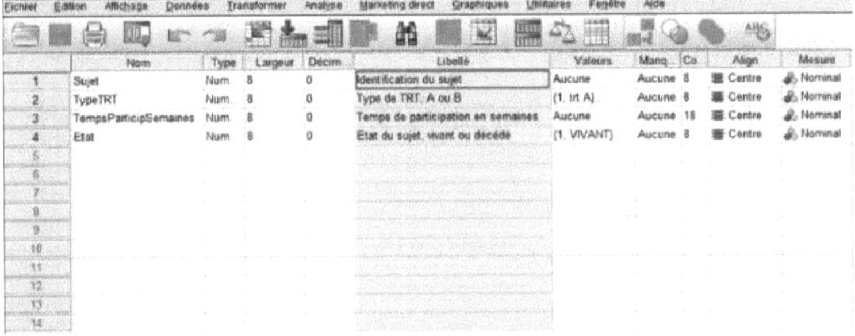

Data presentation

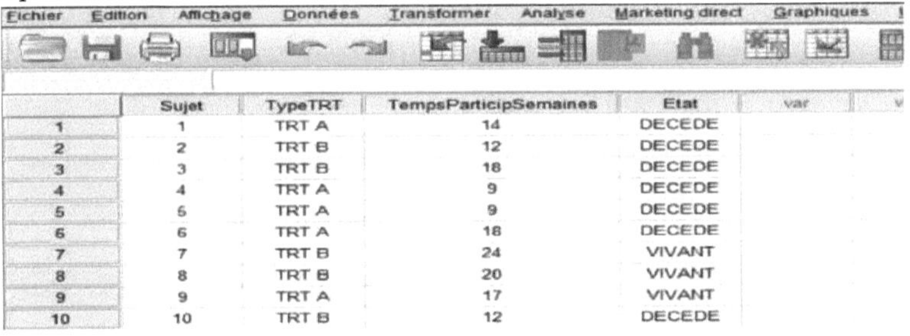

Click on **Analyse > Survie > Kaplan-Meier...** in the main menu, as follows shown below:

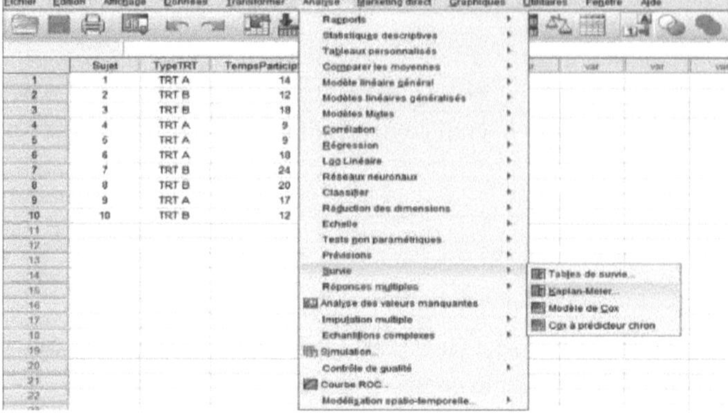

Enter the variables (participation time, subject status and type of TRT) in the spaces (Time, Status and Factor) respectively.

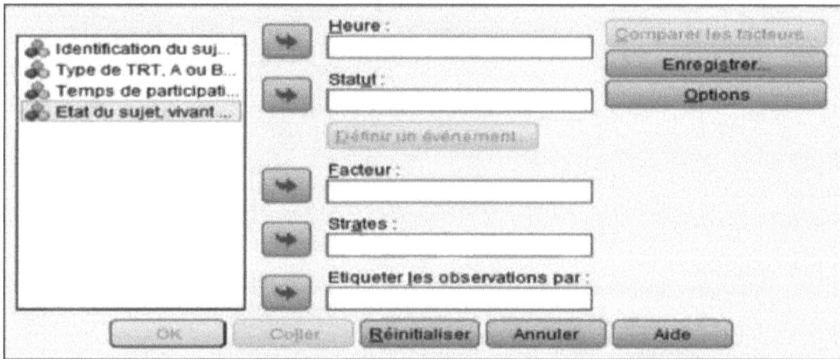

Define the event in the **Status** variable, here the event was death (code 2). Check **Survival** before clicking 'Continue' then **Ok** :

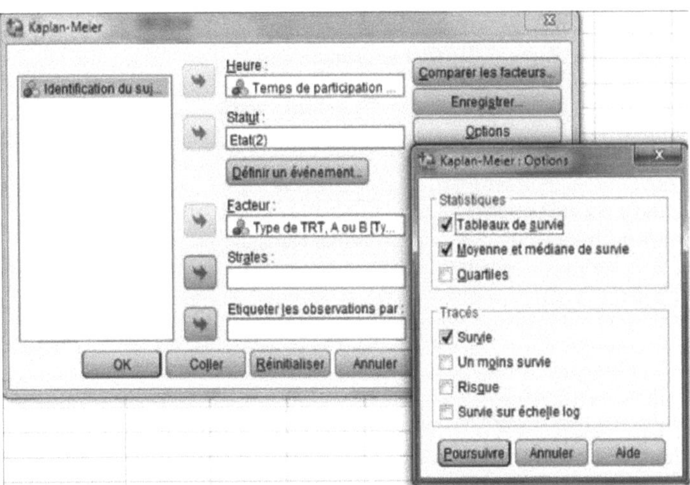

SPSS results:

Survival table						
Type of TRT, A or B	Time	Status	Cumulative survival rate at that time		Cumulative number of events	Number of remaining observations
			Estimate	Standard error		
TRT A	1	9,000	DECEASED	.	.	1	4
	2	9,000	DECEASED	,600	,219	2	3
	3	14,000	DECEASED	,400	,219	3	2
	4	17,000	LIVING	.	.	3	1
	5	18,000	DECEASED	,000	,000	4	0
TRT B	1	12,000	DECEASED	.	.	1	4
	2	12,000	DECEASED	,600	,219	2	3
	3	18,000	DECEASED	,400	,219	3	2
	4	20,000	LIVING	.	.	3	1
	5	24,000	LIVING	.	.	3	0

Compare the two survival curves:

Global comparisons			
	Chi-square	ddl	Sig.
Log Rank (Mantel-Cox)	1,161	1	0,281

Test д'ёда111ё survival distributions for different levels of TRT Type, A or B.

Survival curve for treatments A and B :

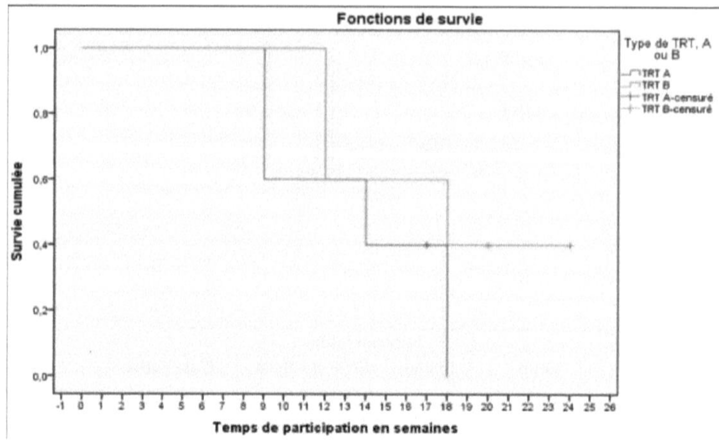

VI. Simple linear regression

Regression is concerned with expressing one variable as a function of another variable. Linear regression is a particular aspect of correlation.

But this can be transformed into a regression situation when we are interested in the changes that affect the first variable when the second variable changes, or vice versa.

If we are interested in variations in weight as a function of age, age is the independent or predictor variable and weight is the dependent or predicted variable.

In other words, we want to predict the value of the **dependent variable** from the **value of** an **independent variable**.

1. Conditions of use

• Normal distribution: the values of the dependent variable are normally distributed. Homogeneity of variances: the variance in the distribution of the dependent variable must be constant for all the values of the independent variable.

• If there is a perfect linear relationship between a predicted variable y and a predictor variable x, in this situation there would be no particular problem in predicting with certainty any value of y as a function of any value of x. All we need to do is apply the equation y = ax +b. This line has an equation of the form

$$\hat{y} = bx + a.$$

• It is customary to write **y = ax + b** in mathematics for perfect relations and y = bx + a in statistics for regression lines. The 'hat' on y only indicates that the predicted variable is y.

2. The equations of the regression lines

The method that best fits a regression line to the point cloud is called the "least squares method". The resulting line is called the 'least squares line'. It is a line such that the sum of the squares of the deviations of the points in the cloud from this line is minimal.

Vertical segments (y as a function of x) and horizontal segments (x as a function of y) are not the same.

The problem, once again, is not that of a strict relationship between the two variables, where the value of one of the two variables can be predicted from the value of the other by means of a single equation.

However, the two regression lines have in common the point which has the mean of x as its abscissa and the mean of y as its ordinate.

The two regression lines form an angle which is smaller the larger the correlation coefficient.

This angle is zero if the relationship between the two variables is strict ($r = \pm 1$), with the two lines forming a single straight line.

The angle between the two lines is 90° if there is a total absence of relationship between the two variables ($r = 0$).

The regression equation for y as a function of x has the expression :

$$\hat{y} - m_y = rs_y/s_x \, (x - m_x).$$

The regression equation for x as a function of y has the expression :

$$x' - m_x = rs_x/s_y \, (y - m_y).$$

In both equations :
- r is the correlation coefficient between x and y ;
- m_y is the average of y ;
- m_x is the average of x ;
- s_y is the standard deviation of y ;
- s_x is the standard deviation of x.

In the expression of the equation of y as a function of x, the slope is:

$$b = rs_y/s_x.$$

Example:

Let's take the data on the distribution of 16 children according to age x and weight y.

The data required to establish the regression equations are:

$$m_x = 10.19 \; ; \; m_y = 34.81 \; ; \; s_x = 2.83 \; ; \; s_y = 11.67 \; ; \; r = 0.91.$$

The equation of the regression line expressing y as a function of x is:

$$\hat{y} - m_y = rs_y/s_x \, (x - m_x)$$

$$\hat{y} - 34.81 = 0.91*11.67/2.83 \, (x - 10.19)$$

$$\hat{y} = 3.75x - 3.43$$

(Using an electronic calculator equipped with a suitable programme, the raw data can be used to calculate : $\hat{y} = 3.76x - 3.47$).

The regression coefficient 3.76 means that weight increases (or decreases) by 3.76 kg when age increases (or decreases) by 1 year.

The equation of the regression line expressing x as a function of y is:

$$x' - m_x = rs_x/s_y\,(y - m_y)$$

$$x' - 10.19 = 0.91*2.83/11.67(y - 34.81)$$

$$x' = 0.22y + 2.51$$

The regression coefficient 0.22 means that age increases (or decreases) by 0.22 years when weight increases (or decreases) by 1 kg.

Consider the regression of weight y as a function of age x and try to predict the mean value of weight for children aged 14. By applying the equation of the corresponding regression line, we find :

$$\hat{y} = 3.75x - 3.43 = 3.75*14 - 3.43 = 49.07.$$

3. SPSS application

- Regression, where we are interested in expressing one variable as a function of another variable, is a particular aspect of correlation.
- We saw in the section on correlation how to measure the relationship between two continuous variables.
- We will now look at how to predict one continuous variable from another.
- We will also look at how best to represent **the linear relationship** between two variables using a mathematical equation;

A. Null hypothesis

In the case of regression, the null hypothesis is that there is no relationship between the dependent variable and the independent variable.

B. Conditions of use

Normal distribution: the values of the dependent variable are normally distributed.

Homogeneity of variances: the variance in the distribution of the dependent variable must be constant for all values of the independent variable.

C. SPSS procedure

- To run a regression, choose **Analyse**,
- then **Regression** and **Linear**,
- Click on . ![arrow] to insert the dependent variable in the box

Dependant and the **independent variable**(s) in their box.

- Since you're doing a simple regression, you only need to place one.
- You also leave the default analysis method, i.e. the **Input** model, which uses all the selected variables to predict the dependent variable.

To proceed with the analysis, click on OK

The button Statistiques...

■ In simple linear regression, you can keep the default statistics provided by SPSS.

■ Firstly, you will obtain the **estimates of** the **regression coefficients** which allow you to reconstruct the equation of the regression line.

■ You will also obtain a table based on the F distribution, giving you information about the **goodness of fit of** the model.

■ Click on Poursuivre to return to the main dialogue box.

- **The** Diagrammes... **button** allows you to create several graphs which can help you to verify certain premises of the regression.

D. SPSS steps :

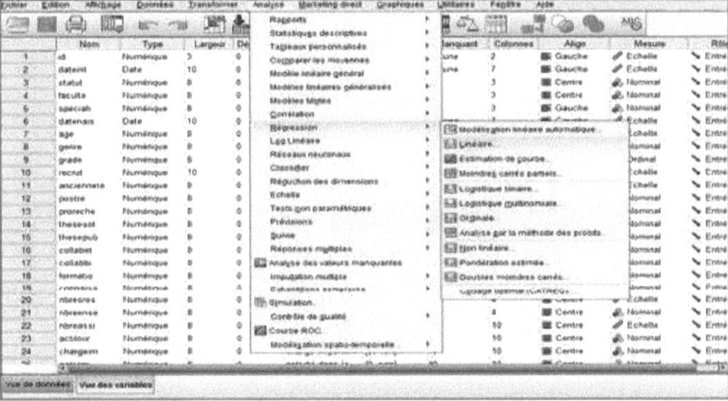

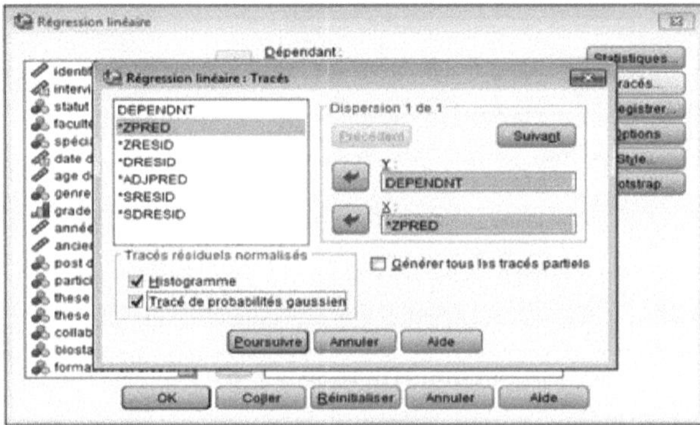

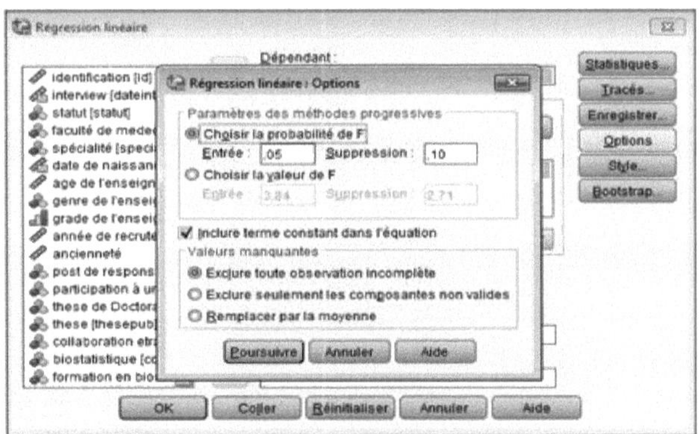

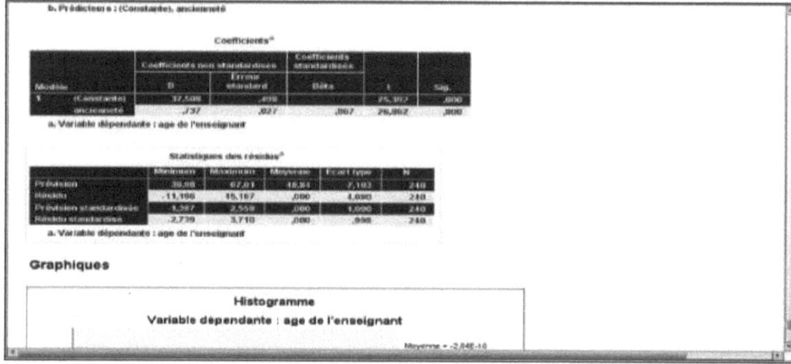

Regression equation y = bx + a

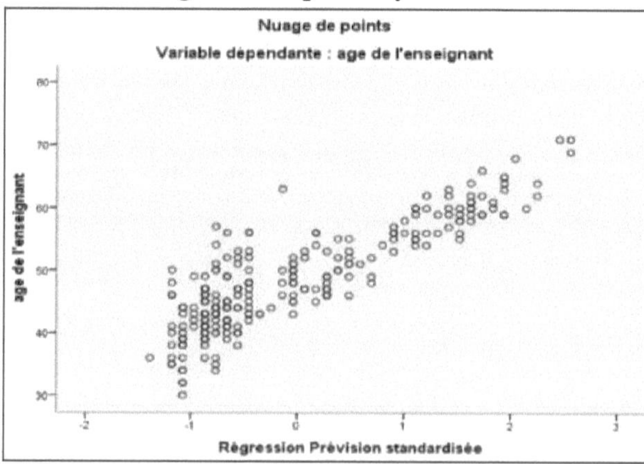

VII. Comparison of several variances

1. Position of the problem

We are sometimes faced with the problem of knowing whether several samples have all been taken from a population with the same variance. In this case, we are comparing several variances.

A number of statistical tests can be used to solve this problem, including **Levene's test (on SPSS),**

The **Bartlett test (**applies to several samples of unequal size, is *very sensitive to the non-normality of* the data in the populations), the **Hartley test** (on equal samples) and the **homogeneity test using the approximate method** (the advantage of using this test is that it is quicker to carry out than the Bartlett test and allows samples of unequal size to be used (impossible in the case of the Hartley test).

2. Levene's test (for homogeneity of variances)

Levene's Test is a statistic used to evaluate the equality of variance for a variable calculated for two or more groups.

H0: the population variances are equal ("**homogeneity of variance**" or "**homoscedasticity**").

If the p-value resulting from Levene's test is less than 5%, it is concluded that there is a difference between the variances in the population from which we have extracted our samples.

A. Example

Let's look at the data in the table below, showing the length of hospitalisation in days for three groups of accident victims.

Table : Breakdown of three groups of accident victims according to length of hospitalisation in days

Route	9		4	14	10	15	2	8	55	5	30	30	7	12
Drop	19		3	6	45	11	10	2	4	3				
Foreign bodies	1		2	1	2	4	3	7	16					

We want to know whether the three samples are all taken from a population of the same S^2.

Database :

Step 1: Click on **Analysis > Compare means > 1-factor ANOVA >** in the main menu, as shown below:

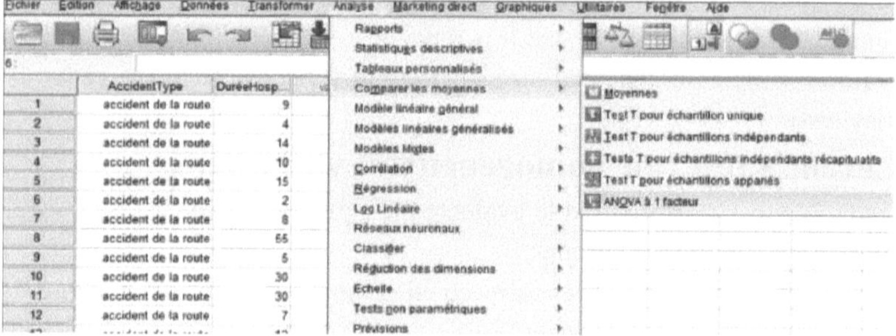

Step 2: After entering the two variables '**Duration of hospitalisation**' and '**Type of accident**' in the '**List of dependent variables:**' and '**Factor**' spaces respectively, click on the '**Options**' button.

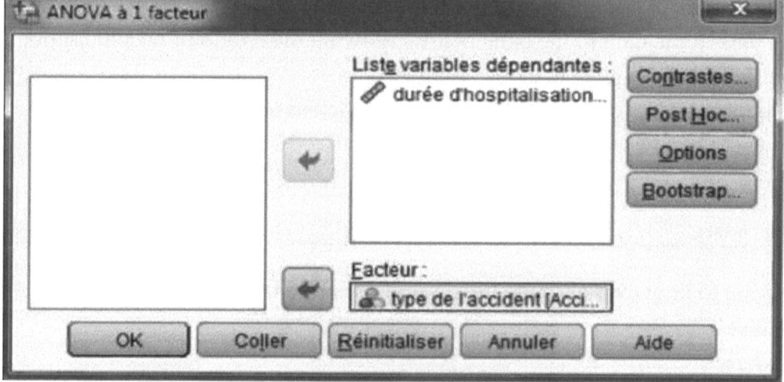

Step 3: After clicking on '**Options**' you will be presented with the following dialog box, tick the '**Variance homogeneity test**' and click on '**Continue**' after '**OK**':

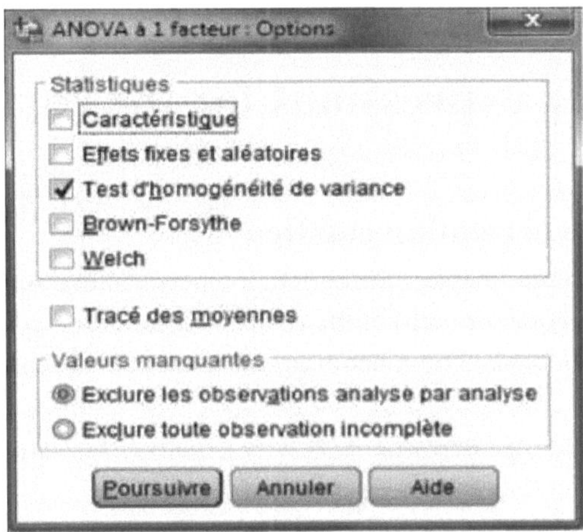

Step 4: After clicking on 'OK', you will be presented with the following results:

Variance homogeneity test

length of hospitalisation in days

Levene statistics	ddl1	ddl2	Sig.
1,730	2	27	.196

ANOVA

length of hospitalisation in days

	Sum of edges	ddl	Medium square	F	Sig.
Inter-group	595,214	2	297,607	1,868	.174
Intragroup	4301,453	27	159,313		
Total	4896,667	29			

Significance of results: The three samples do not come from a population with the same variance *(p = 0.196)*.

VIII. Other expressions for the correlation coefficient

1. Spearman correlation coefficient: r'

This coefficient is used to assess the correlation between two sets of ranks. This is useful when one (or both) of the characteristics observed cannot be measured but can be ranked (number of injuries, number of deaths in our example).

This coefficient is always between **-1** (strictly negative correlation) and **+1** (strictly positive correlation).

The following examples are taken from the textbook **'Tests statistiques en sciences medicales'**.

Example: table **11.2 p 141**: the following data relate to the number of people injured and killed in road accidents in 16 wilayates.

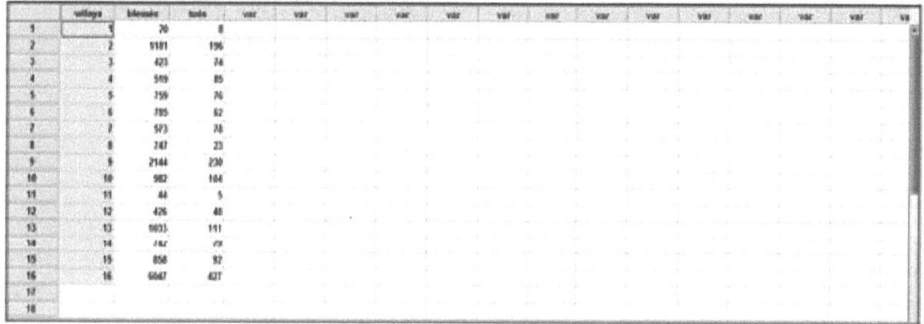

Step 1: Click on **Analyse > Correlation > Bivariee...** in the main menu, as shown below:

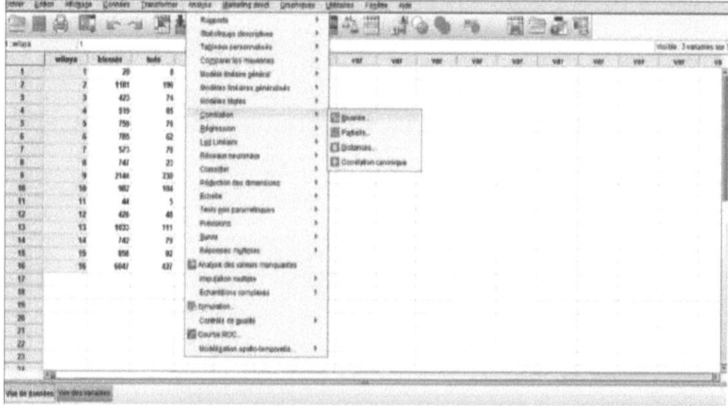

Step 2: Once you have selected the two variables **'number of deaths'** and **'number of injuries'** and entered them in the **'variables'** space, choosing the **Spearman test**, you will see the dialog box below:

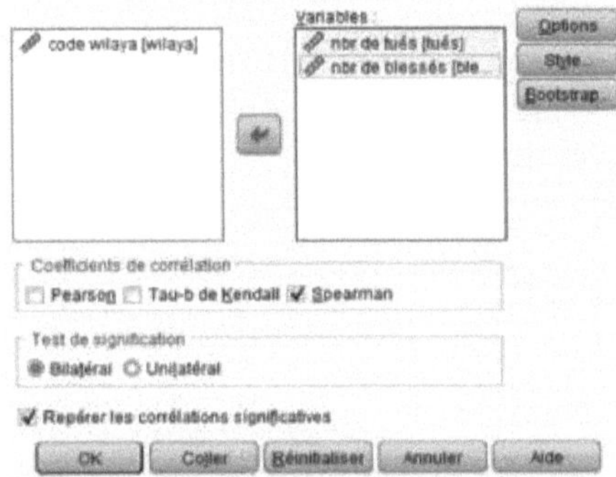

Step 3: Click on 'ok' to get the following results:

	Number of kills	Number of injuries
Rho of number of Correlation coefficient Spearman tues Sig (bilateral) N	1,000 . 16	,856 ,000 16
Number of Correlation coefficient injuries Sig (bilateral) N	,856 ,000 16	1,000 . 16

Meaning of results:
There is a significantly (<0.001) positive correlation (+ 0.86) between the number of injuries and the number of fatalities, and it can also be said that the number of injuries tends to increase (or decrease) when the number of fatalities increases (decreases).

2. Bi-serial point correlation coefficient: rpb

This coefficient is a special expression of the Bravais Pearson r coefficient. It expresses the correlation between a dichotomous variable **of nature 'x'** and a quantitative variable 'y'.

The rpb coefficient is always between **-1** (strict negative correlation) and **+1** (strict positive correlation).

Let's consider the following data, in which we are trying to establish a possible correlation between a dichotomous variable 'x' with two modes (1 = male, 0 = female) and a quantitative variable 'y' (physics marks/25) from 10 pairs of data.

Student	Sex of student	Physics grade /25
1	Male	9
2	Female	10

3	Female	14
4	Male	19
5	Male	17
6	Male	15
7	Female	7
8	Male	20
9	Male	25
10	Female	6

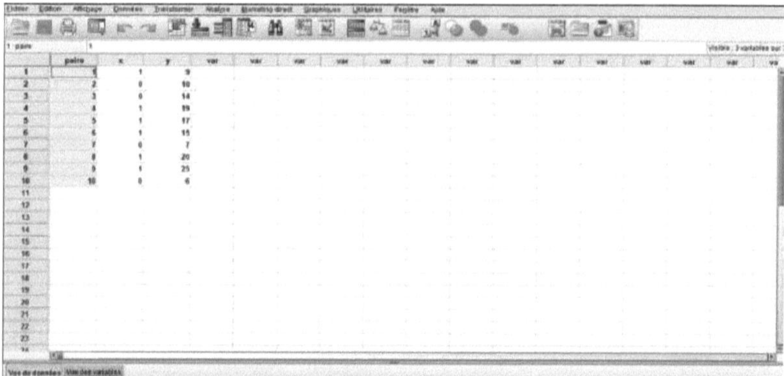

Step 1: Click on **Analyse> Correlation > Bivariee...** in the main menu, as shown below:

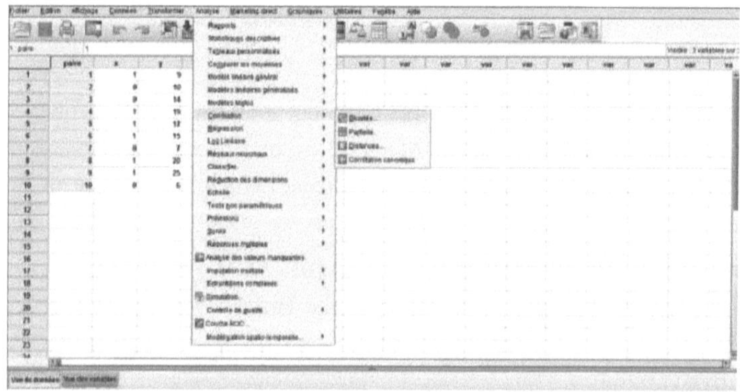

Step 2: After selecting the two variables **'physics grade/25'** and **'student's gender'** and entering them in the **'variables'** area, choose the **Bravais Pearson test.** The dialog box below will appear:

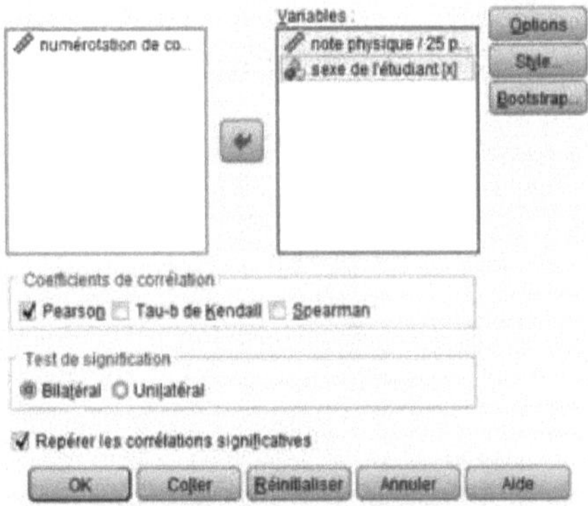

Step 3: Click on 'ok' to obtain the following results:

	physical score / 25 points	gender of student
Physical score / 25 Pearson correlation points Sig. (bilaterale) N	1 10	,688* ,028 10
Sex of studentPearson correlation Sig. (bilaterale) N	,688* ,028 10	1 10

*. The correlation is significant at the 0.05 level (bilateral).

Meaning of result:

There is a significantly (0.028 < 0.05) positive correlation (+ 0.69) between the gender of the student and the physics grade.

3. Quadruple correlation coefficient or phi coefficient: rf

This coefficient can be calculated for both independent and matched samples, and is used to assess the correlation between two dichotomous variables.

A. Example 1:

Table 11.7 p 152: results of treatments A and B on two samples pairs (148 pairs)

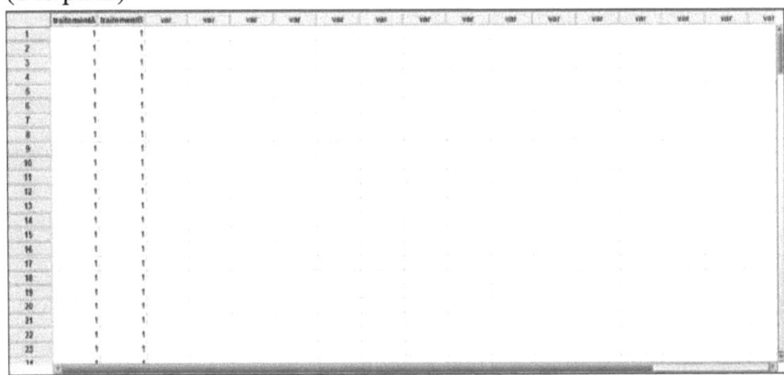

Step 1: Click on **Analyse> Descriptive statistics > Crosstabs** in the main menu, as shown below:

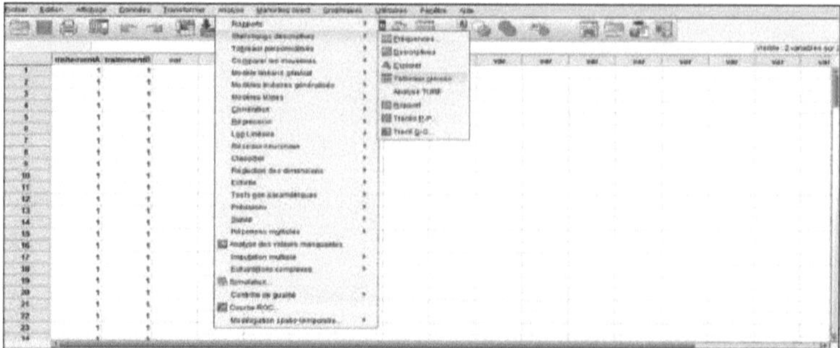

Step 2: After entering the two variables in the '**row'** and '**column'** spaces and clicking on the '**statistics'** button, choose the '**phi and v of cramer'** test in the '**nominal'** space. The dialogue box below will appear:

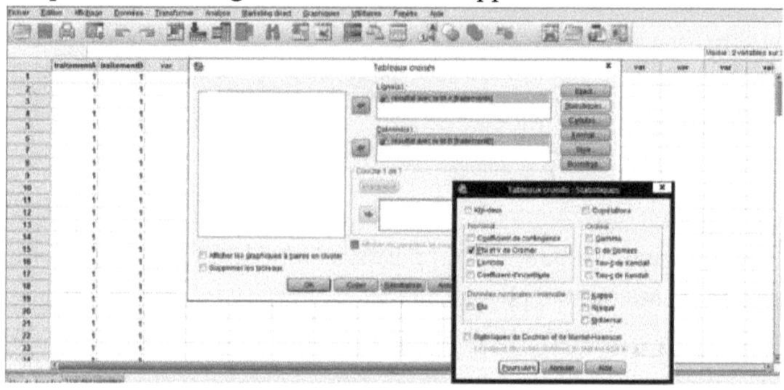

Step 3: Click on 'ok' to see the following results:

Cross table result with TRT B * result with TRT A

		Results with TRT A		
		Failure	Success	**Total**
Results with TRT B	Failure	50	20	70
Success		9	69	78
	Total	59	89	148

McNemar Chi-square = 3.45 p = 0.063

	Value	Approximate meaning
Nominal per Phi Nominal	,611	,000
V de Cramer	,611	,000
N of valid observations	148	

Meaning of result:

There is a significant correlation between the results generated by the two treatments. Individuals tend to respond in the same way to both treatments (if successful with treatment A, often successful with treatment B). We would have had a negative phi coefficient if the patients had responded in opposite ways to the two treatments.

B. Second example:

Table 11.8 p 153: results of two treatments A and B on two paired samples (29 pairs).

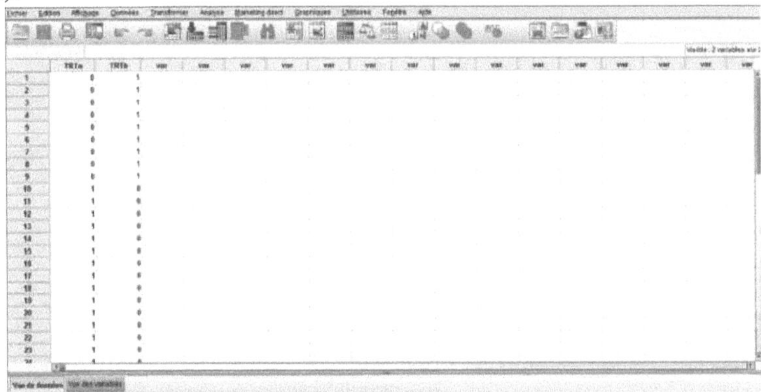

Follow the same steps as the first example

Cross table result with treatment B * result with treatment A

	Results with treatment A		Total
	Failure	Success	
Result with treatment B Failure	0	20	20
Success	9	0	9
Total	9	20	29

Chi-square tests

	Value	Sig. exacte (bilaterale)
Test of Mc Nemar		,061·
N of valid observations	29	

	Value	Approximate meaning
Nominal per Phi Nominal	-1,000	,000
V de Cramer	1,000	,000
N of valid observations	29	

Meaning of result:

There is a significantly negative correlation between the results generated by the two treatments. Individuals did not tend to respond in the same way to the two treatments (if successful with treatment A, often unsuccessful with treatment B and vice versa). The phi coefficient was strictly negative because the patients had responded in strictly opposite ways to the two treatments.

71

C. Example 3:

DEMS 2019 (Schwartz): two sleeping pills A and B were administered to 14 insomniac subjects. The subjects received A once and B once, in random order. Sleep times are reported in the following database:

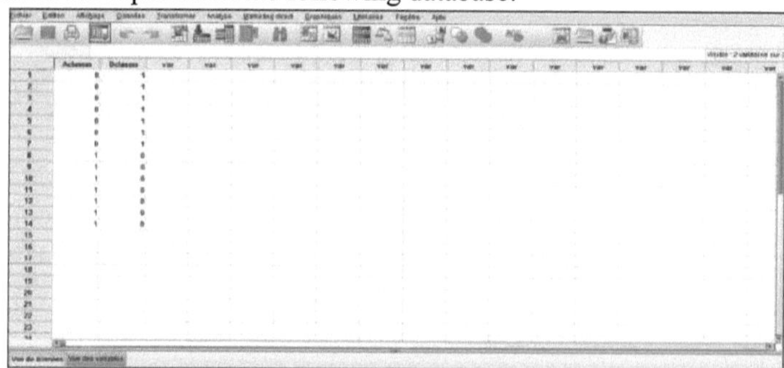

Follow the same steps as the first example

Cross table result with treatment A * result with treatment B

	Results with treatment B: success, failure		
	Failure	Success	**Total**
Result with treatment Failure A: success, failure	0	7	7
Success	7	0	7
Total	7	7	14

Chi-square tests

	Value	Exact Sig. (bilateral)
Test of Mc Nemar		1,000·
N of valid observations	14	

Symmetrical measurements

	Value	Approximate meaning
Phi	-1,000	,000
Nominal per Nominal V de Cramer	1,000	,000
N of valid observations	14	

Meaning of result:

There was a significantly (p<0.001) negative correlation (phi = -1) between the results generated by the two treatments.

Individuals do not tend to respond in the same way to the two treatments (if successful with treatment A, often unsuccessful with treatment B and vice versa).

The phi coefficient was strictly negative (-1) because the patients had responded in strictly opposite ways to the two treatments.

4. Pearson's C contingency coefficient

This coefficient evaluates the correlation between two variables in a contingency table where *at least* one of *the two variables has more than two modes*.

We can say that the C coefficient measures the degree of association between two qualitative variables.

In the following example, we have two categorical variables, one with three modes (social class) and the other with two modes (infected and non-infected). Let's take the data from **table 3.1 p 44** (prevalence of a viral infection according to social class) in the following database:

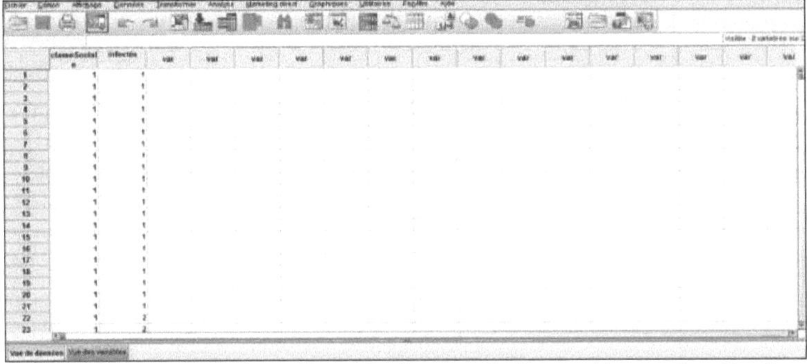

Step 1: Click on **Analysis > Descriptive statistics > Crosstabs.** In the main menu, as shown below:

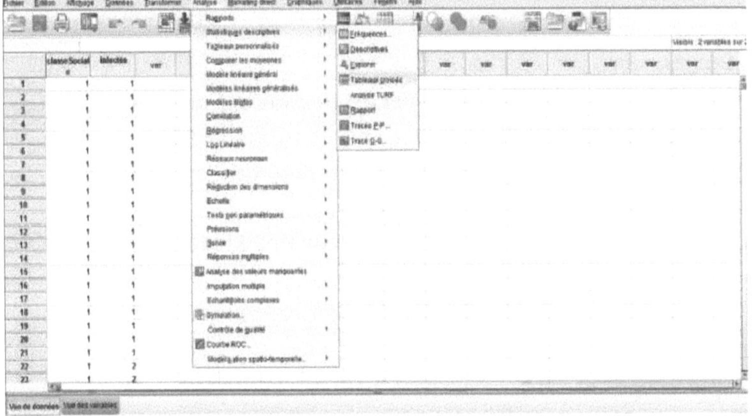

Step 2: After entering the two variables in the **'row'** and **'column'** boxes and clicking on the **'statistics'** button, choose the **'contingency coefficient'** in the **'nominal'** box. The dialog box below will appear:

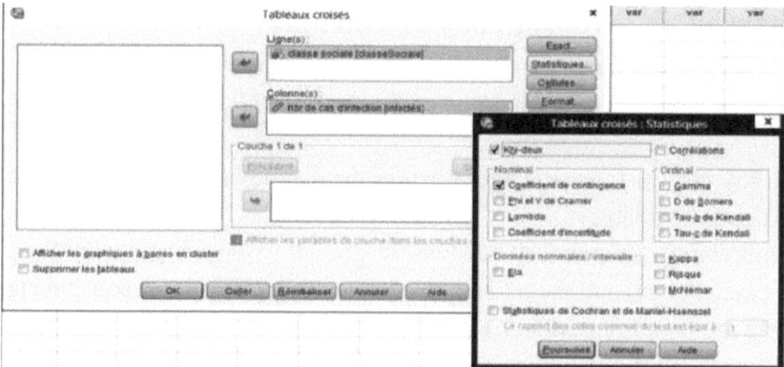

Step 3: click on 'continue' then 'ok' to obtain the following results:

Social class cross-tabulation * number of cases of infection

	Viral infection		Total
	Yes	No	
Social class Favourite	21	191	212
Average	141	857	998
Defavorisee	62	230	292
Total	224	1278	1502

Symmetrical measurements

	Value	Approximate meaning
Nominal by NominalCoefficient of contingency	,096	,001
N of valid observations	1502	

Meaning of results:

The result (C = 0.096) measures the degree of co-occurrence (link) between the nominal dependent variable (Y = infection with two modalities) and the nominal independent variable (X = social class with more than two modalities) in our sample.

• Remember that if C = 0, there is no correlation, whereas if C = 1, there is a perfect link between X and Y.

• By convention, we will say that the relationship between X and Y is:

■ **Perfect,** if the value of **C = 1.**

■ **Very strong,** if **C > 0.8.**

■ **Strong,** if C is between **0.5 and 0.8.**

■ **of average** intensity, if C is between **0.2 and 0.5.**

■ **Low,** if C is between **0 and 0.2.**

■ **Nil,** if **C = 0**

In our example C = 0.096 with a p = 0.001, this means that there is a **significant** link between viral infection and social class, but this link is **weak**.

NB: this contingency coefficient C can be calculated differently:

$C = \sqrt{[X^2/(X^2 + n)]}$, $X^2 = 13.86 \Rightarrow C = \sqrt{[13.86/(13.86+ 1502)]} = \mathbf{0.0956}$

	Value	ddl	Asymptotic significance (bilateral)
Pearson chi-square	13,864ᵃ	2	,001
Likelihood ratio	13,461	2	,001
Association line by line	13,317	1	,000
N of valid observations	1502		

a. 0 cells (0.0%) have a theoretical size of less than 5. The minimum theoretical size is 31.62.

5. Kendall's W concordance coefficient

Kendall's concordance coefficient **W is** designed to evaluate the correlation between several sets **k** of **n** ranks.

Consider the data in table **11.9 on page 158,** which classifies **10 wilayates** according to the number of cases reported for **4** fecal peril **diseases** (cholera, typhoid fever, viral hepatitis A, dysentery).

The wilaya ranked first has the highest number of cases reported, while the one ranked tenth has the lowest.

The question is whether the ranks assigned to the wilayates for each disease are consistent or, in other words, whether the rankings for each disease are consistent.

This coefficient only takes positive values, if **W = 0** expresses **total discordance** between the k sets of n ranks while **W = 1** expresses **perfect agreement**.

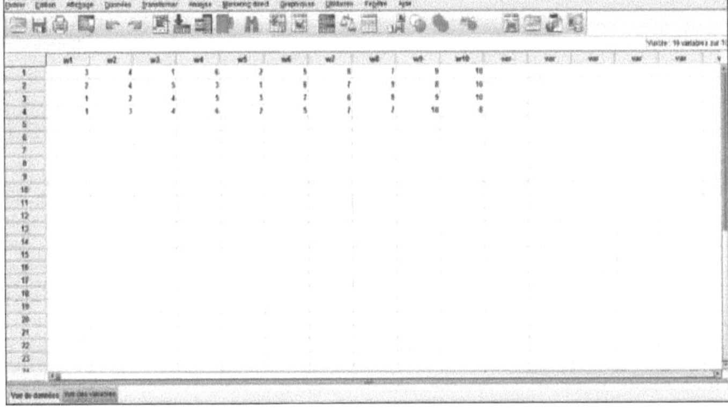

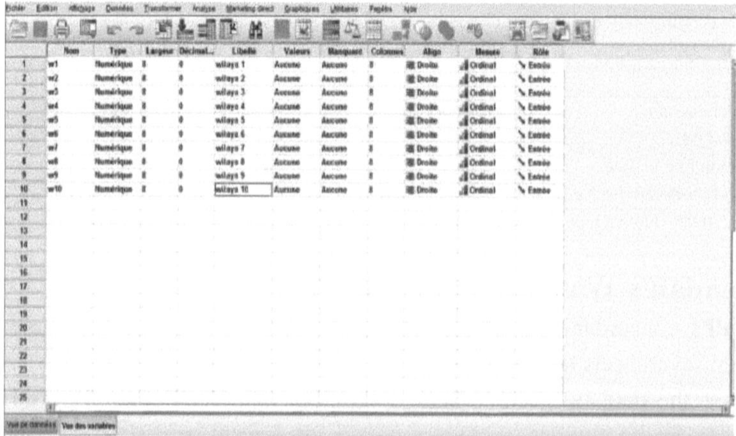

Step 1: Click on **Analyse> tests non parametriques > boite de dialogue ancienne version > K echantillons lies.** In the main menu, as shown below :

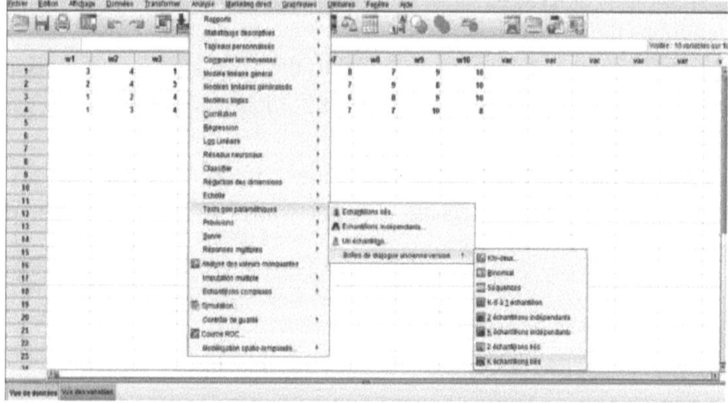

Step 2: Once you have entered all the variables in the **'variables to be tested'** space, choose **Kendall's W concordance coefficient** in the **'test type'** space. The dialog box below will appear:

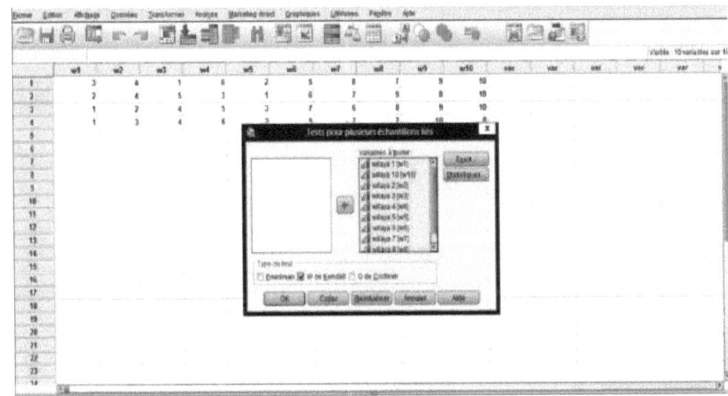

Step 3: Click on 'ok' to see the following results:

Wilaya	Average rank
wilaya 1	1,75
wilaya 2	3,25
wilaya 3	3,50
wilaya 4	5,00
wilaya 5	2,00
wilaya 6	5,75
wilaya 7	7,13
wilaya 8	7,88
wilaya 9	9,00
wilaya 10	9,75

Statistical tests

N	4
W de Kendall	,902
Chi-square	32,463
ddl	9
Meaning	,000

Meaning of result:

The ranks occupied by the wilayates for each faecal peril disease tend to be identical.

When a wilaya is badly classified (or well classified), it is classified for all fecal peril diseases.

This agreement is significantly strong *(p <0.001, w = 0.9).*

IX. Correlation between two quantitative variables

1. Correlation

In general terms, the correlation technique concerns the study of the relationship between two variables, taking into account the fact that they are measured on the same observation unit.

* The unit in question may be a healthy subject or a sick subject,
* In a correlation situation, each of the two variables is considered to be dependent, and the aim is to identify any link between them.

2. SPSS procedure

* Correlation can be found in the **Analysis** menu, under **Correlation**.
* Choose **Bi variee,** correlation between two variables.
* Partial correlation takes into account a control variable.
* In the main dialogue box, use the arrow to insert
* Continuous variables to be tested in the **Variable** box ;
* You can choose between three correlation coefficients:

1. **Pearson** (default): coefficient calculated for continuous variables
2. **Kendall's tau-b** and **Spearman**: these tests are non-parametric measures. (The coefficient is calculated for ordinal categorial variables).

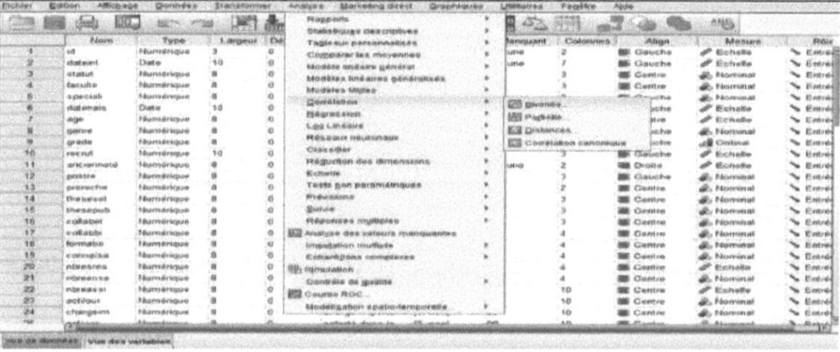

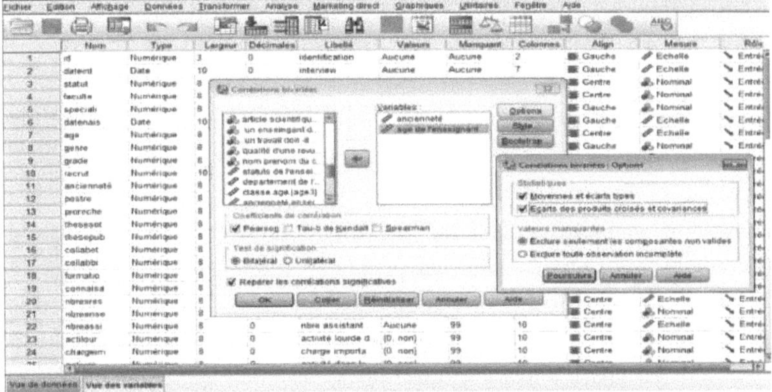

- You can then determine the type of hypothesis test to be verified,
- If the research hypothesis clearly indicates the direction of the association, you can choose the unilateral test, otherwise leave the default option of the bilateral test.
- You also leave the option **Mark significant correlations** ticked so that SPSS can highlight them with asterisks.

- Then click on 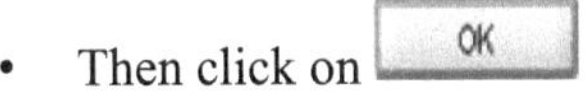

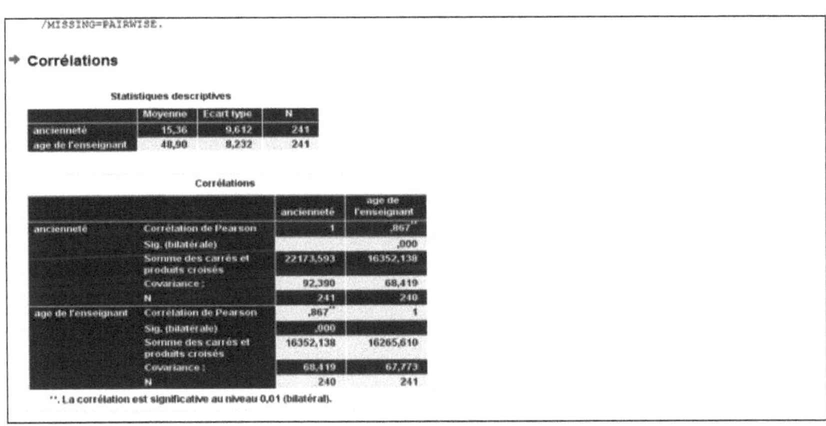

Correlation result :

The correlation table is fairly **simple to interpret**. It is a cross-tabulation between the variables that are related.

In each box representing the crossing of two variables, we can see the value of the coefficient accompanied by asterisks if the correlation is significant, the associated degree of significance and the number of observations that have been crossed.

Since correlation is a symmetrical measure, we can see that the coefficient is the same for the association between **age and seniority** and for the association between seniority and age.

3. Correlation results

Terms and conditions :

Linearity condition :

* It must be emphasised that the Bravais-Pearson correlation coefficient r applies only to linear relationships between two variables.
* In fact, a non-significant correlation does not necessarily imply the absence of a relationship, it only implies the absence of a linear relationship.
* To assess whether the relationship is linear, as a first approximation we can construct the scatter diagram and consider the cloud of points.

Assumption of homoscedasticity and normality of distributions :

* The assumption of equal variability in the conditional distributions of y for each value of x and vice versa.

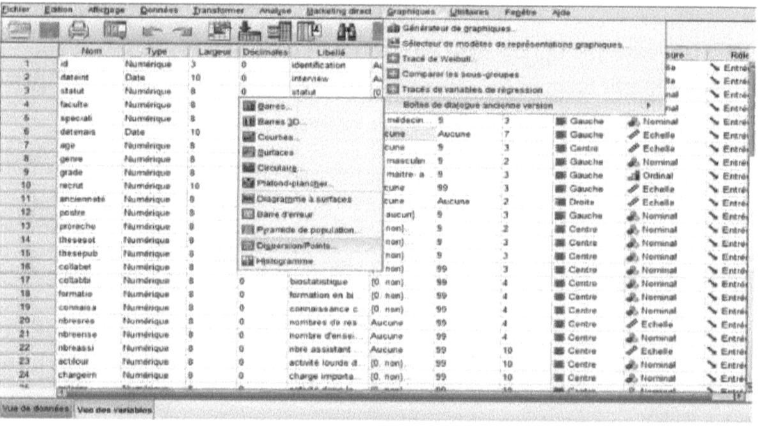

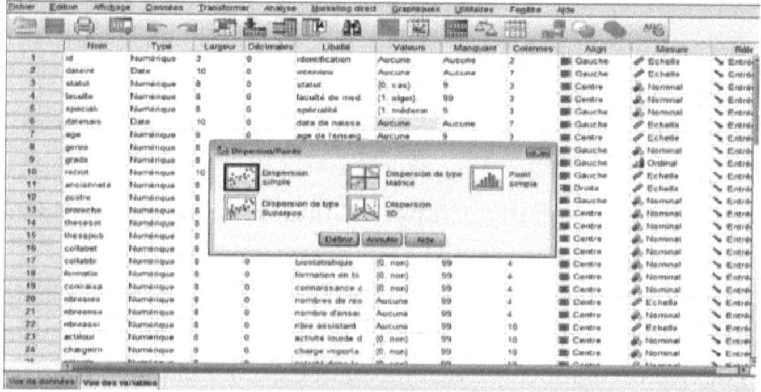

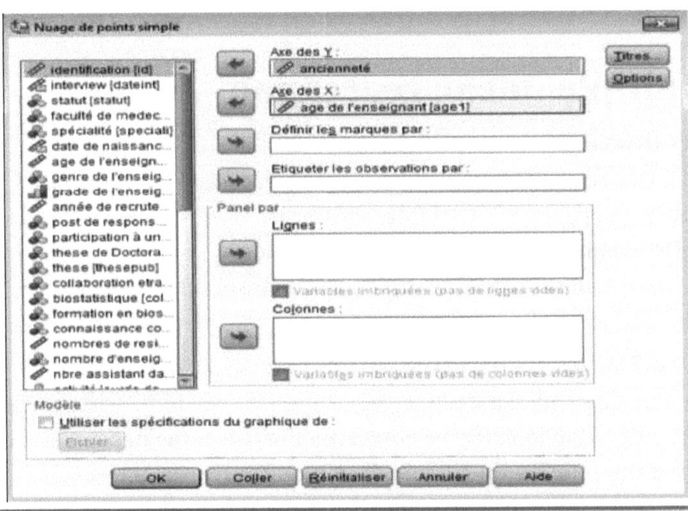

Nuage de points simple
identification [id]
interview [dateint]
statut [statut]
faculté de medec...
spécialité [speciali]
date de naissanc...
age de l'enseign...
genre de l'enseig...
grade de l'enseig...
année de recrute...
post de respons...
participation à un...
these de Doctora...
these [thesepub]
collaboration etra...
biostatistique [col...
formation en bios...
connaissance co...
nombres de resi...
nombre d'enseig...
nbre assistant da...
Axe des Y :
ancienneté
Axe des X :
age de l'enseignant [age1]
Définir les marques par :
Etiqueter les observations par :
Panel par
Lignes :
Variables imbriquées (pas de lignes vides)
Colonnes :
Variables imbriquées (pas de colonnes vides)
Titres...
Options...
Modèle
Utiliser les spécifications du graphique de :
Fichier...
OK   Coller   Réinitialiser   Annuler   Aide

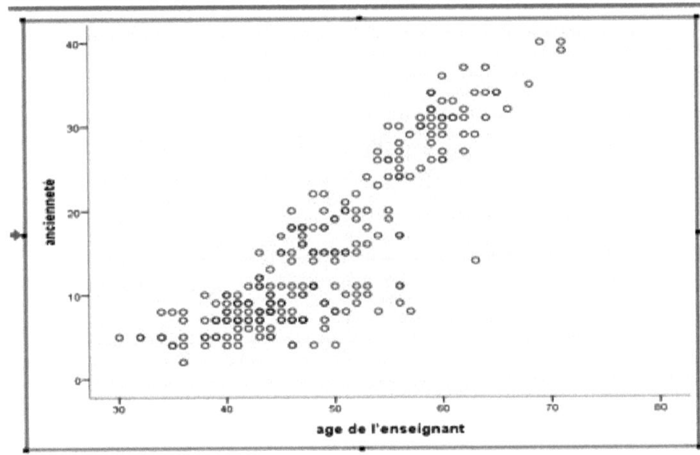

ancienneté
age de l'enseignant

X. Multiple linear regression

1. Introduction

Multiple linear regression is a multivariate technique used when faced with **a quantitative dependent variable** (glycated haemoglobin HbA1c) and **supposedly explanatory, quantitative independent variables** (age, history of diabetes, waist circumference, systolic blood pressure, blood cholesterol, body mass index and microalbuminuria).

2. Correlation or causality bivariate analysis

Before proceeding with the multivariate analysis, it would be wiser to carry out a bivariate analysis to look for the **correlation between the dependent variable and each of the supposedly independent explanatory variables.**

A bivariate analysis involves studying the relationship between 2 variables:

- Are they related?
- Do the values of one influence the values of the other?
- Or are they, on the contrary, independent

The variable under influence is called the dependent variable.

The variable which produces the effect is called the independent variable.

- What type of analysis to choose
- The method of analysis to be chosen according to the nature of the variables.

The following table summarises the application of the tests in the bivariate analysis

		Explanatory variable X	
Variable Y to be explained		**Quantitative** Linear regression	**Qualitative** One-factor analysis of variance Chi-square test of independence
	Quantitative	Simple correlation	
	Qualitative	Logistic regression	

Correlation: Make a scatter plot: X and Y are interchangeable Calculation of correlation coefficient = COV(x,y)/ecart-standard(X) * ecart-standard(Y)

Decision board to study l'association

- *1st step: calculating the Pearson coefficient r :* The Pearson coefficient is an index reflecting a linear relationship between two continuous variables.

A **positive** sign indicates that the 2 variables are moving in the same direction.

A **negative** sign indicates that the 2 variables vary in opposite directions.

- *2nd step: definition of the null hypothesis:* The value of r obtained is an estimate of the correlation between two continuous variables in the population. Its value will therefore fluctuate from one sample to another. We therefore want to know whether, in the population, these two variables are really correlated or not. We therefore need to carry out a hypothesis test.

H0: No correlation between the two variables H1: Correlation between the two variables.

- *Calculating the critical probability (p-value):* The SPSS software proposes the critical probability (p-value), which must be compared with the risk a that we set (1% or 5%). If the p-value is smaller than a , then we reject the null hypothesis.

3. Multiple linear regression

This is a method of analysing quantitative data, the aim of which is to study the causality between a particular variable known as the quantitative explained variable and other explanatory variables.

The algebraic model :

A. Steps to take to analyse multiple linear regression

1. Estimation of regression coefficients „...
2. Measuring the quality of the model, the R2 (coefficient of determination).
3. To check whether the marginal contribution of each variable Xi to the explanation of Y is significant.
4. Choice of the optimal model and discussion of the results with the literature.

B. Estimation of coefficients

The criterion chosen to estimate the regression coefficients, in the context of an MLR, is always the same as in the case of simple MLR: the ordinary least squares method.

By minimizing the sum of the squares of the errors (residues) between the explained variable Y and the sum We obtain the least squares estimates , ...and .

C. Goodness of fit GOF

R2 coefficient of determination or percentage of variance explained by regression

Properties:

- Allows you to judge the quality of the regression
- Ideal = 1
- Bad regression = 0

D. Is the link significant overall?

Model :

Fisher hypothesis test :

- H0: (Y = does not depend on X)
- H1: At least one (Y depends on at least one X)

Statistics used: $\rightarrow$ F(p,n-p-1)

- F Fisher's law with (p,n-p-1) degree of freedom: f value with probability

0.05 of being exceeded.

- Rejection of H0 if Fc>F-tabule.

E. Is the marginal contribution of each variable significant?

Model :

Student's t test:

- H0: (Xi can be deleted)
- H1: (Xi must be retained.

Statistics used :

- Decision: to reject H0 at the risk of being wrong: rejection of H0 if t calculates > in absolute value to t tabulates.

F. Test for collinearity between independent variables :

- It is necessary to test for collinearity, as multiple collinearity between explanatory variables biases the estimates of R2 ;
- Tolerance is required: percentage of the explanatory variable not explained by the other variables.
- Tolerance (xj)=1-R2 (it must be close to 1, and in any case >0.3)we also need to study the VIF (variance inflation factor): VIF +1/tolerance
- Degree of increase in error due to multi-colinearity (the VIF must be less than 4).

4. Procedure in SPSS

Dataset :

	HbA1c	Age	Ancienneté	Tourtaille	PAS	Cholesterol	IMC	Microalb	sexe
1	14.7	37	1	128	120	2.59	34.3	10.0	
2	6.5	58	5	97	140	2.15	27.5	17.0	
3	10.8	79	10	100	140	1.50	27.1	35.0	
4	5.4	38	0	133	130	1.81	53.7	28.0	
5	10.9	63	8	85	140	1.73	27.3	61.0	
6	6.8	56	6	93	130	1.85	25.3	145.0	
7	6.2	48	4	85	130	2.30	27.1	12.0	
8	9.2	72	2	91	130	1.53	24.5	16.0	
9	12.6	56	8	87	120	2.12	24.1	9.0	
10	6.4	58	1	100	140	1.77	34.1	23.0	
11	6.0	73	7	110	120	1.25	33.0	11.0	
12	9.6	52	0	100	140	1.72	31.1	11.0	
13	6.8	66	21	106	140	1.87	26.8	5.0	
14	5.7	49	6	80	120	1.48	33.6	6.0	
15	8.7	40	9	140	120	1.57	48.2	7.0	
16	7.9	68	11	96	161	1.00	29.3	25.0	
17	8.7	52	0	94	140	2.29	30.8	7.0	
18	6.7	69	10	96	143	1.66	25.5	32.0	
19	5.9	70	3	99	140	2.03	32.6	68.0	
20	6.0	64	1	100	130	1.41	32.2	18.0	
21	7.4	72	14	96	170	2.36	27.0	19.0	
22	6.3	63	14	40	170	2.01	20.8	300.0	
23	5.6	47	0	121	130	1.90	43.8	50.0	
24	10.3	58	17	40	120	1.17	32.3	18.0	
25	11.6	66	3	106	150	2.41	33.2	79.0	
26	6.7	57	10	80	110	1.18	22.5	8.0	
27	7.7	67	8	61	150	2.58	25.8	10.0	

Under SPSS: Analysis $\rightarrow$ Linear regression (input method)

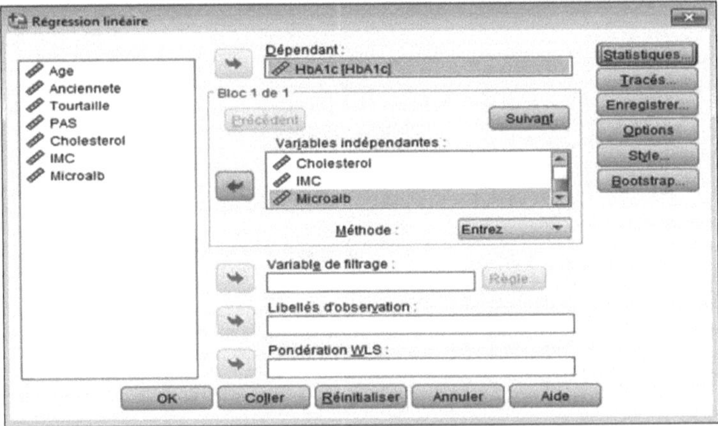

In statistics: choose :
- Estimation, Goodness of fit
- Durbin-Watson test: to check the independence of the residuals, we
generally check that this statistic is between 1.5 and 2.5.

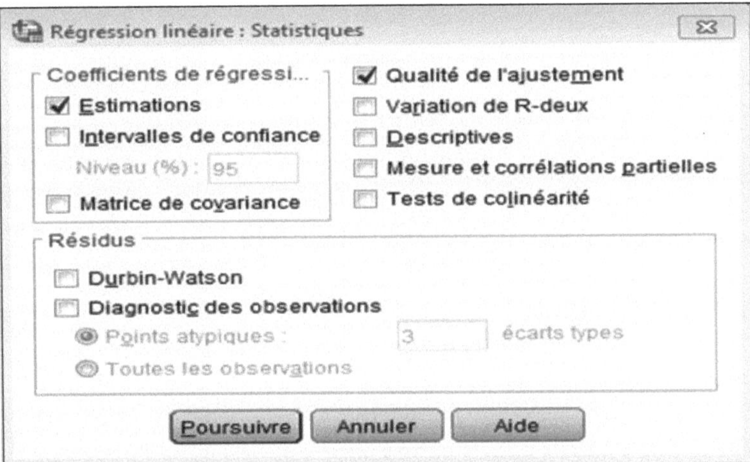

In tracks:
- To find the residue normality graphically :
o histograms to check the normality of residues graphically
o Gaussian probability traces: which allow a graphical appreciation between an observed distribution and a theoretical model.
- Homoscedasticity of residuals to be checked graphically by plotting

standardised residuals against predicted y values.

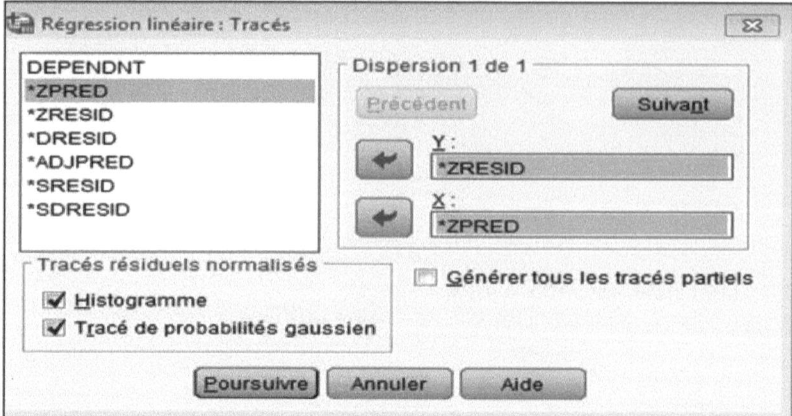

In Save: tick :

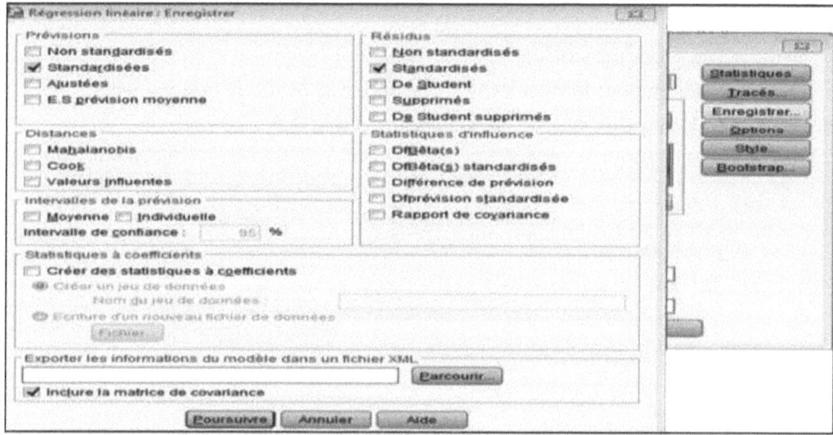

In option: leave as default

Output:

Table: Variables introduced into the model

Variables introduced/eliminateda

Model	Variables introduced	Variables eliminated	Method
1	Microalb, BMI, Cholesterol, Old age, PAS, Age	.	Enter

a. Dependent variable : HbAlc

b. All the variables requested have been introduced.

Model summary[b]					
Model	R	R-two	R-two adjusts	Standard error of the estimate	Durbin- Watson
1	,299[a]	,090	,063	1,7192	2,092

a. Predictors: (Constant), Microalb, BMI, Cholesterol, Tourtaille, Anciennete, PAS, Age
b. Dependent variable : HbA1 c

Interpretation:

- *The R-two* represents the proportion of variability explained by the model in relation to the total variability. Here, it is low and represents only 2.99% of the total variability.
- *The coefficient R^2* [R^2 = 1- (SCR/SCT)] measures the fit of the model to the data. It increases as the number of variables included in the model increases. It can be used to compare models with the same number of variables.
- *The adjusted R-two* (more reliable than the R^2) [$R\ j^2_{aus\ te}$ =1- (SCR/(n-p-1))/(SCT/n-1))] estimates the R^2 in the population, independently of the number of variables. It does not necessarily increase when the number of variables introduced into the model increases. It can be used to compare models with a different number of variables.
- *The Durbin-Watson test is* used to test the independence of the residuals. In general, we check that this statistic is between 1.5 and 2.5 (which is the case here).

ANOVA table :

ANOVAa

Model	Sum of edges	ddl	Medium square	F	Sig.
1 Regression	69,820	7	9,974	3,375	,002[b]
Residu	709,353	240	2,956		
Total	779,173	247			

a. Dependent variable : HbA1c
b. Predictors: (Constant), Microalb, BMI, Cholesterol, Tourtaille, Anciennete, PAS, Age

Since the significance of the model tested is less than 0.05, the null hypothesis of no link between the variables can be rejected.

- The statistic of F=3.375 exceeds the critical value in Fisher's table at 7 and 247 ddl, for a significance level of 5%.
- By comparing the associated significance of 0.002 with the significance level, we reach the same conclusion, namely that the regression is highly significant.

Coefficients

Model	Non-standardised coefficients		Standardised coefficients	t	Sig.	95.0% confidence interval for B		Colinearite statistics	
	B	Standard error	Beta			Lower terminal	Top terminal	Tolerance	VIF

Model		B	Standard error	Beta	t	Sig.	Metered bollard	Top terminal	Tolerance	VIF
1	(Constant)	6.651	1.290		5,155	.000	4,109	9,192		
	Age	.022	,011	-,137	-1,968	,050	-.045	,000	,787	1,271
	Old	.046	,015	.209	3,101	,002	,017	.075	,837	1,195
	Tourtaille	.017	.006	,196	3,016	,003	,006	,027	,898	1,114
	NOT	,001	,006	,014	.217	,829	-.011	,014	,858	1,166
	Cholesterol	,358	.249	,092	1,444	,150	-.131	,850	,939	1.066
	BMI	-.015	,022	-.044	-.663	.508	-.059	,029	,857	1,166
	Microalb	,001	,001	,033	,493	,623	-.002	,003	,870	1,149

a. Dependent variable HbA1 c

- The non-standardised coefficient corresponds to the model's b coefficients. They measure the effects of the independent variables on the dependent variable. As the units of measurement are not the same for all the variables, a simple technique for obtaining standardised coefficients consists of centring and reducing all the variables and running a regression on the transformed data (the standardised coefficient).

- The student test for age (sig. = 0.05) and PAS (sig. = 0.829), cholesterol (sig. = 0.150), BMI (0.508) and Microal(sig. = 0.623) are not included in the explanation of Y, so the H1 hypotheses for these variables are not valid ^ The regression must be repeated.

- Once the variable with the smallest contribution to the model has been removed if the change in R^2 is not significant, it is eliminated. The procedure will be repeated until all the variables retained contribute significantly to the improvement in R^2 .

Modele 2 (modele 1- PAS) : We start with PAS p-value = 0.8 the highest and we will look at the significance of the model:

ANOVAa

Model	Sum of edges	ddl	Medium square	F	Sig.
1 Regression	69,681	6	11,614	3,945	,001ᵇ
Residu	709,492	241	2,944		
Total	779,173	247			

a. Dependent variable : HbAlc

b. Predictors: (Constant), Microalb, BMI, Cholesterol, Tourtaille, Anciennete, Age

Coefficients

Model		Non-standardised coefficients		Standardised coefficients	t	Sig.	95.0% confidence interval forB		Colinearite statistics	
		B	Standard error	Beta			Metered bollard	Top terminal	Tolerance	VIF
1	(Constant)	6,788	1,123		6.042	.000	4.575	9,000		
	Age	-,022	,011	-,134	-1,965	.051	-.044	,000	,815	1,227
	Old	,046	,015	,209	3,113	.002	,017	,075	,837	1,194
	Tourtaille	,017	,005	,i&-	3,038	.003	,005	,027	,901	1,110
	Cholesterol	,367	,246	.094	1,492	.137	-.118	,852	,957	1,045
	BMI	-.015	,022	-.044	-.660	.510	-.058	,029	,858	1.166
	Microalb	,001	.001	,036	.571	,569	-.002	,003	,934	1,071

a dependent variable: HbA1 c

Model 2 is still significant, so we continue to remove the significant variables one by one.

Model 3 (model 2-microalb): p-value of t test = 0.569

ANOVAa

Model	Sum of edges	ddl	Medium square	F	Sig.

Model	Sum of edges	ddl	Medium square	F	Sig.
1 Regression	68,723	5	13,745	4,682	,000ᵇ
Residu	710,451	242	2,936		
Total	779,173	247			

a.   Dependent variable : HbAlc

b.   Predictors: (Constant), BMI, Cholesterol, Old age, Tourtaille, Age

Coefficients

Model	Non-standardised coefficients		Standardised coefficients	t	Sig.	95% confidence interval for B		Statistiques by colin9arlt9	
	B	Standard error	Beta			Lower terminal	Top terminal	Tolerance	VIF
1 (Constant)	6.746	1.118		6.026	.000	4,540	8.951		
Age	-,021	,011	-,130	-1,922	,066	-.043	.001	,823	1,216
Old	.048	.015	,216	3.288	,001	.019	.076	.869	1,150
Tourtaille	.017	.005	,198	3,055	,003	.006	,027	.901	1,110
Cholesterol	.377	.245	,096	1.538	,125	-.106	.860	.962	1,040
BMI	-.014	.022	-.043	-,646	.519	-.058	.029	.858	1,165

a. Dependent variable: HbAlc

Model 3 still significant Fisher p-value less than 0.05

Model 4: model 3 - BMI :

ANOVAa

Model	Sum of edges	ddl	Medium square	F	Sig.
1 Regression	67,496	4	16,874	5,762	,000ᵇ
Residu	711,677	243	2,929		
Total	779,173	247			

a.   Dependent variable : HbAlc

b.   Predictors: (Constant), Cholesterol, Age, Tourtaille, Age

Coefficients

Model	Non-standardised coefficients		Standardised coefficients	1	Sig.	95.0% confidence interval for B		Colinearite statistics	
	B	Standard error	Beta			Lower terminal	Top terminal	Tolerance	VtF
1 (Constant)	6,348	,934		6,797	.000	4,508	8,187		
Age	-.020	,011	-.122	-1.839	.067	-.041	.001	,849	1,178
Old	,049	,014	,222	3,397	.001	,021	,077	,883	1,133
Tourtaille	,016	,005	,185	3,003	.003	,005	,026	,991	1,009
Cholesterol	,371	,245	.095	1.517	.131	-,111	,853	.963	1,039

a. Dependent variable: HbA1 c

Fisher test still significant

Student's t test cholesterol NS ^ remove variable cholesterol and repeat the analysis

Model 4: model 3 - CHOL

ANOVAa

Model	Sum of edges	ddl	Medium square	F	Sig.
1 Regression	60,755	3	20,252	6,878	,000ᵇ
Residu	718,418	244	2,944		
Total	779,173	247			

a.   Dependent variable : HbAlc

b.   Predictors: (Constant), Tourtaille, Anciennete, Age

Coefficients

Model	Non-standardised coefficients		Standardised coefficients	t	Sig.	95.0% confidence interval for B		Statistics for colineante	
	B	Standard error	Beta			Lower terminal	Top terminal	Tolerance	VIF
1 (Constant)	7,217	,740		9,756	.000	5.760	8.674		
Age	-.023	.011	<140	-2.139	,033	-.044	-.002	,877	1,140

| Old | .049 | .014 | .223 | 3,415 | .001 | .021 | .076 | .883 | 1.133 |
| Tourtaille | .015 | .005 | .1181 | 2,936 | .004 | | .005 .025 | .993 | 1,007 |

a Dependent variable: HbA1 c

In the end, we adopted model 4: with age, age and size as explanatory parameters.

5. Verification of the chosen model hypothesis

A. Check that there is no multi-collinearity between the variables, in 2 possible ways

The tolerance or VIF is calculated:

- Tolerance = $1 - R^2$; The VIF (variance inflation factor) is the inverse of the tolerance.

- Tolerance = $1 - R^2$ (Portion of the variance of the variable that is not explained by the other explanatory variables: must be greater than 0.1 or VIF < 10)

Coefficients[a]

Model	Non-standardised coefficients		Standardised coefficients	1	Sij).	95.0% confidence interval for B		Colinearite statistics	
	B	Standard error	Beta			Internal bollard	Top terminal	Tolerance	VIF
1 (Constant)	7,217	,740		9,756	,000		5,760 8.674		
Age Old Tourtaille	-,023	,011	-,140	-2,139	,033		-.044 -.002	,877	1,140
	,049	,014	,223	3,415	,001	,021	.078	,883	1,133
	,015	,005	.181	2.936	,004		,005 .026	,993	1,007

a. variable dependants : HbA1 c

The result is consistent with the absence of multi-collinearity between the variables.

B. Residue assumption

Residue normality is checked graphically using a histogram or PP-plot.

Histogram:

- The following graph shows the normality of the standardised residuals. Remember that the standardised residual follows a reduced centred normal distribution.

- As the graph shows, the average is close to 0, and the majority of values are between -2 and +2.

Histogram

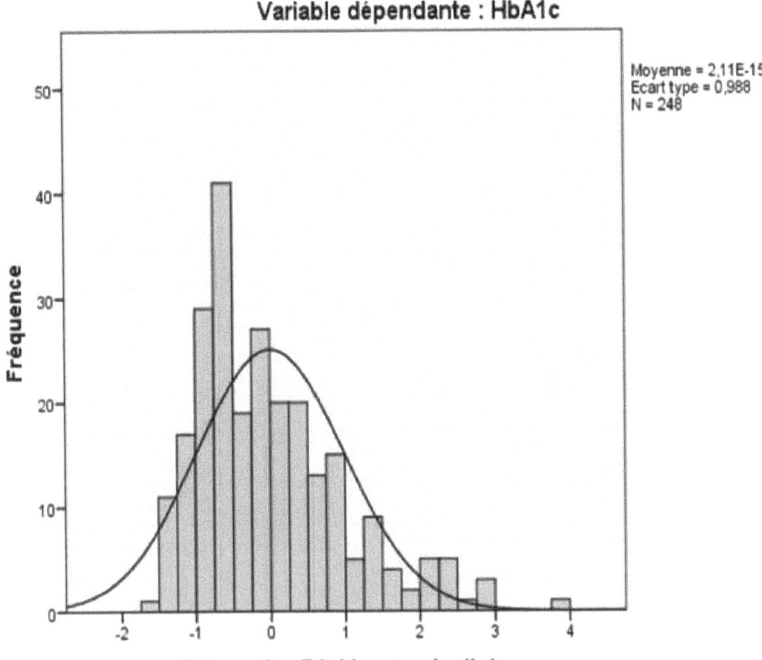

The P-P plot:

It compares the observed distribution with the theoretical distribution (values predicted by the model) and should be located at the 1ere bisector. In the graph below, the ordinate axis shows the cumulative frequencies of the theoretical distribution and the abscissa axis shows the cumulative probabilities of the observed distribution.

The point cloud aligns with the 1ere bisector when the proposed theoretical distribution is a good representation of the observations. Any significant deviations from alignment can be identified and analysed. In this graph, there is a deviation in the intermediate values, where the cumulative frequency of predicted values is lower than the cumulative frequency of observed values.

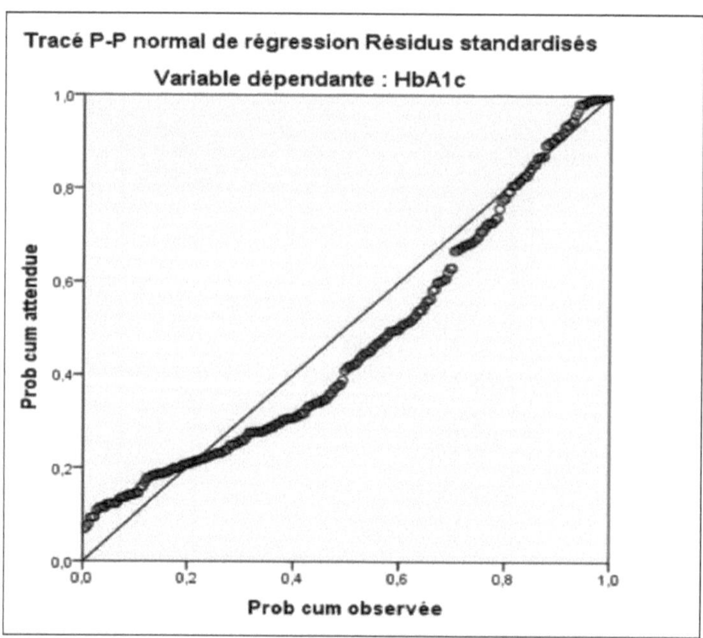

Homogeneity of variances:

It is used when the variance of the residuals does not depend on the value of the predictors, as shown graphically below (no funnel shape):

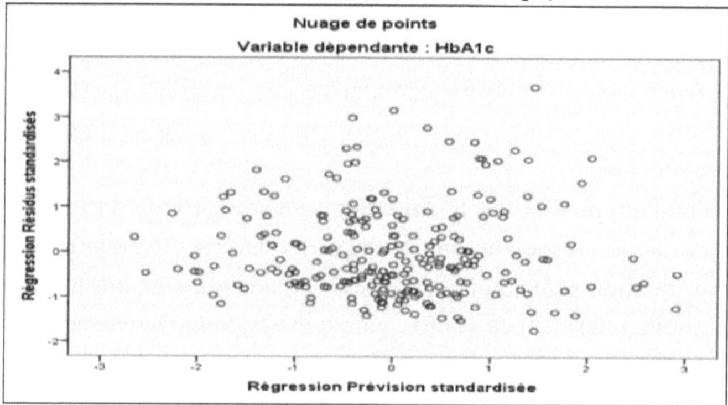

Done the model is written: $y_i = 7.217 + 0.049$ Old $+ 0.015$ Small $+ 0.23$ Age :

- Increasing the age of a measurement unit will increase the dHBlac rate by 0.049, at a constant level for the other variables;
- Increasing the size of the cake by one unit will mean increasing the Hblac rate by 0.015 at a constant level of the other variables;
- Increasing the age of a unit increases the Hblac rate by 0.23 independently of the other variables.

Note: when writing the model: y is predicted as a function of the non-standardised coefficients and are listed in descending order of significance, i.e. starting with the b's with the lowest p-value.

Coefficients[3]

Model	Non-standardised coefficients		Standardised coefficients	t	Sig.	95.0% confidence interval for B		Colinearite statistics	
	S	Standard error	Beta			Lower terminal	Top terminal	Tolerance	VIF
1 (Constant)	7,217	.740		9,756	.000	5.760	8,674		
Age	-.023	.011	-,140	-2,139	,033	-.044	-,002	,077	1.1 40
Old	.049	,014	,223	3,415	.001	,021	,07B	,803	1.1 33
Tourtaille	.015	.005	.181	2,935	.004	,005	,026	,993	1.007

a. Dependent variable: HbAt c

We start with *intercept*, then *old*, then *tourtaille* and finally *Page*.

XI. Analysis of variance by factorial design

1. Introduction

The analysis of variance with a factorial design is as follows: Linear model analysis ^ general ^ univariate :

- A quantitative explanatory variable (Hemoglobin A1c)
- 2 qualitative explanatory variables :

o Anc diab = Age grouped into 4 classes (< 5; from 5 to 9; from 10 to 19; >20)

o Obad (or abdominal obesity) grouped into 3 classes (waist circumference < 88; from 88 to 101; > 102)

Put in dependent variable : HbA1c and nominal variables as fixed variables

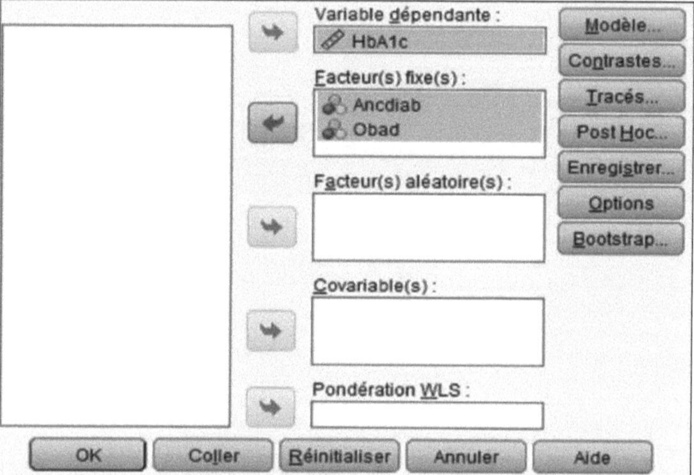

2. Model with interaction

In model:

Leave the default option, i.e. the full factorial model, which includes the effect of all the independent variables and the interaction effect between them. You leave the "Include constant in model" option ticked ^ click Continue :

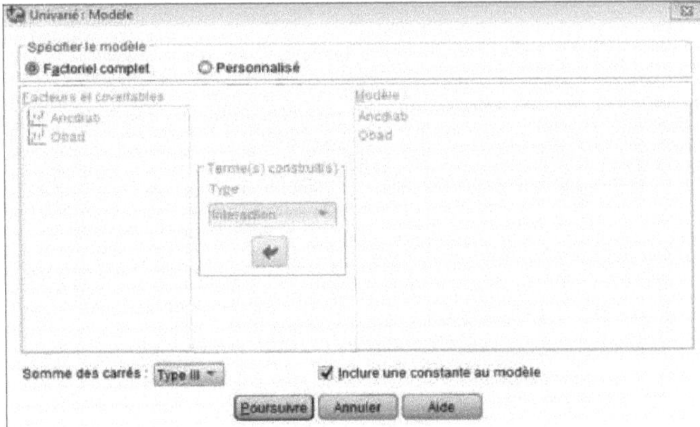

In trace:

This option is really interesting, because it allows you to observe the relationship between the groups in a graph, making it easier to interpret the term interaction.

Put the variable age in the horizontal axis and in the separate curve ^ click on add.

Click on **continue**. The interaction between the two variables should appear in the **diagram** box. Then click on **continue**:

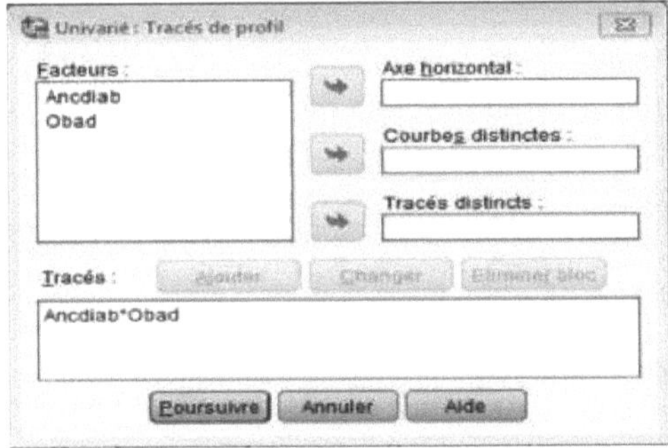

In options :

The first part provides the estimated marginal mean in the population for the entire model (OVERALL), each VI or the interaction between 2 VIs. Transfer all variables :

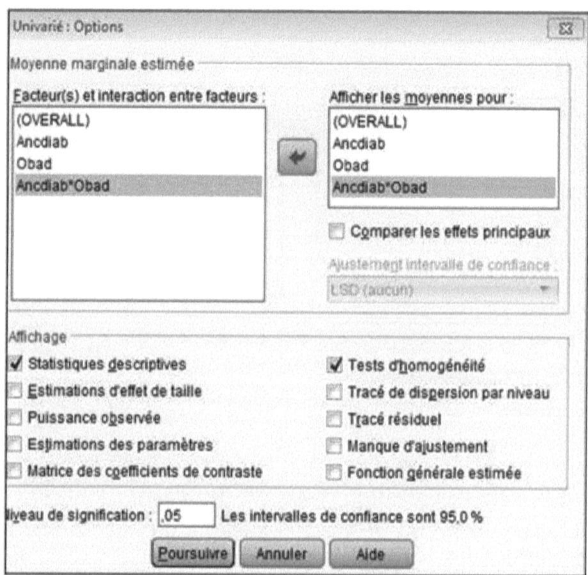

OUTPUT

The 1er table gives the distribution of the numbers for each mode of the nominal variable:

Inter-subject factors

		N
Ancdiab	1	103
	2	62
	3	62
	4	21
Obad	1	72
	2	111
	3	65

The second table shows the descriptive statistics for HbAlc levels as a function of factor modality:

Descriptive statistics

Dependent variable: HbAlc

Ancdiab	Obad	Average	Standard deviation	N
1	1	6,743	1,3733	30
	2	7,238	1,3079	48
	3	7,412	2,1454	25
	Total	7,136	1,5736	103
2	1	7,994	2,2201	18
	2	7,629	1,6924	21
	3	7,622	1,7812	23

	Total	7,732	1,8669	62
3	1	7,556	2,0092	18
	2	8,76	1,5694	30
	3	8,921	2,0242	14
	Total	8,447	1,8718	62
4	1	7,983	1,6726	6
	2	7,475	0,9265	12
	3	8,3	1,9468	3
	Total	7,738	1,2874	21
Total	1	7,363	1,8491	72
	2	7,749	1,5462	111
	3	7,852	2,0302	65
	Total	7,664	1,7761	248

• The 1st column gives the mean HbAlc level in each subgroup, e.g. the mean Hb1Ac level for those with code 3 age and code 3 waist circumference is 6.743% whereas the subgroup with code 1 age and code 2 waist circumference is 7.23%. In total, if we merge the 3 subgroups, we find that the mean Hb1Ac rate for the factor 1 old age category is 7.136.

• The highest mean HbAlc level was found in the group with age code 3 and waist circumference code 3, while the lowest mean HbAlc level was found in the subgroup with age code 1 and waist circumference code 1, with values of 8.92 and 6 respectively.

• In view of the results, there is a difference between the mean HbA1c levels of the samples, but the question to be asked is whether there is a significant difference between the mean HbA1c levels of the populations from which these samples come.

• The $2^{c\;me}$ column gives us the standard deviations for each subgroup, measuring the average dispersion of the variability of the HbA1c levels of N subjects in each subgroup. Is there a statistically significant difference in standard deviations between the different groups?

3. Hypotheses to be tested in ANOVA

A. Variance homogeneity test

• H0 : (homoscedasticity)

• H1: at least 2 groups differ in their variance (heteroscedasticity)

Levene, Bartlett test $(p\;value > \alpha \rightarrow$ H0 not rejected)

Equality of variance test for Levene's errors

Dependent variable: HbAlc

F	ddl1	ddl2	Meaning
1,111	11	236	0,353

Tests the null hypothesis that the error variance of the dependent variable is equal across the different groups.

a. Plan: Constant + Ancdiab + Obad + Ancdiab * Obad

p-value = 0.353 (> 0.05) ^ therefore H0 is not rejected the hypothesis of homosedasecity is retained

B. Normalized HbAlc levels in the groups

In SPSS normality tests are: Kolmogorov Smirnov(KS: for large sample) and Shapiro-Wilk (for small sample).

SPSS procedure:

- Analysis ^ descriptive statistics ^ explore
- In plot: tick plot with test, in Levens test: tick untransformed(we will work on the initial variables).

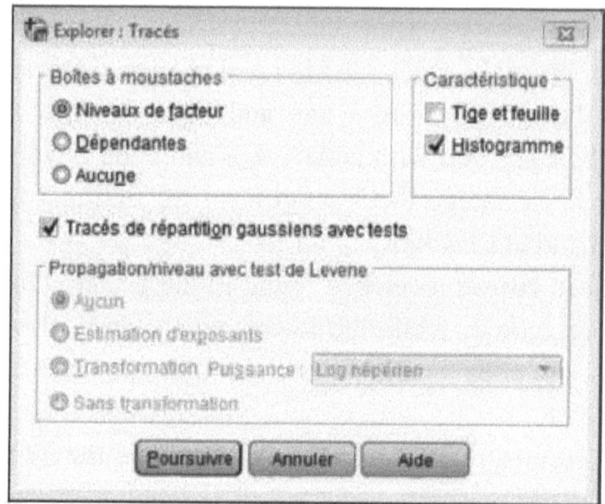

Normality tests

	Kolmogorov-Smirnov a			Shapiro-Wilk		
	Statistics	ddl	Sig.	Statistics	ddl	Sig.
HbAlc	0,126	127	,000	0,918	127	,000

a. Correction of the meaning of Lilliefors

Kolmogorov Smirnov test of normality is significant *(p* value = 0.000) so the normality of the dependent variable is rejected.

This is confirmed graphically:

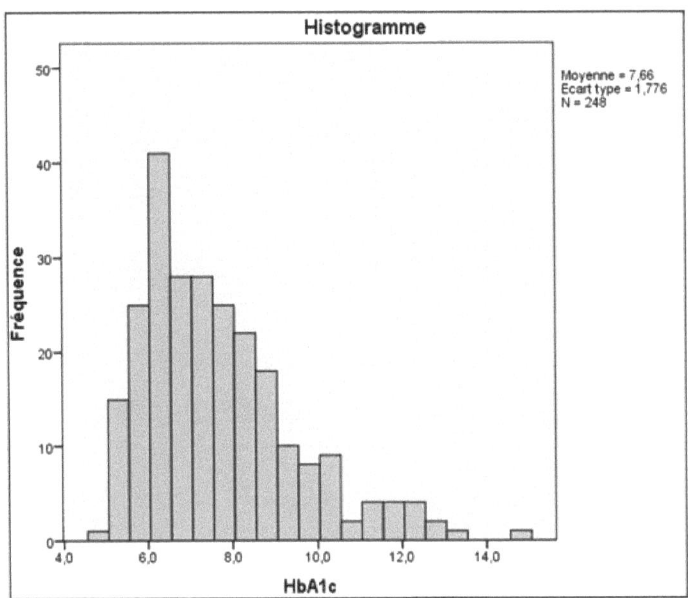

The histogram of the HbAlc distribution is asymmetrical

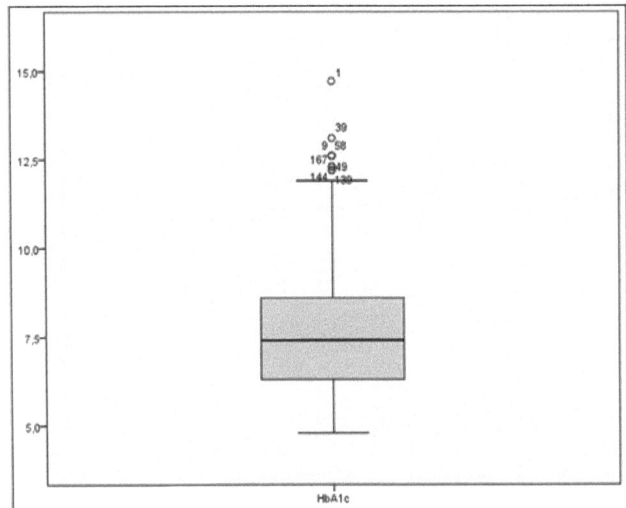

The moustache box confirms the asymmetry of the HbAlc distribution, with the median almost in the middle of the box, but the lengths of the moustaches are disproportionate to the presence of outliers.

4. Search for outliers

Analysis $\rightarrow$ descriptive statistics $\rightarrow$ descriptive ! put VD in variables and tick the standardised variables:

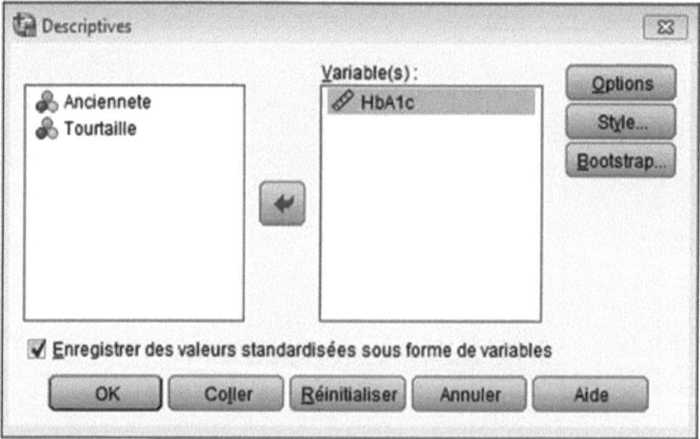

Output: Appearance of Z score :

	HbA1c	Anciennete	Tourtaille	ZHbA1c	var
1	15	1	2	3,55387	
2	13	3	1	2,72420	
3	13	2	1	2,46492	
4	13	2	1	2,46492	
5	12	3	2	2,30936	
6	12	2	2	2,10194	
7	12	3	2	1,99823	
8	12	1	2	1,89452	
9	12	3	2	1,89452	
10	11	3	1	1,84267	
11	11	3	1	1,79082	
12	11	2	1	1,58340	
13	11	3	2	1,53154	
14	10	3	1	1,27227	
15	10	3	2	1,27227	
16	10	1	1	1,22042	
17	10	3	2	1,22042	
18	10	1	1	1,16856	
19	10	1	2	1,06485	
20	10	1	2	1,06485	
21	10	3	2	1,01300	
22	10	1	2	,90929	
23	10	2	2	,85744	

The observation is considered an outlier if Z score > 3 or Z score $< -3 \rightarrow$ presence of an outlier with HbA1c = 15%.

Outliers must be excluded from the analysis.

5. Anova has 2 non-interacting factors

3 hypotheses to test

- effect of age factor

- waist circumference factor
- effect of the interaction age * waist circumference

Note that :
- the interaction term is insignificant > 0.05
- the mean HbAlc level: the mean HbAlc levels differed significantly according to the type of diabetes (p < 0.05), and did not differ significantly according to the age of the diabetes.

Tests for between-subjects effects

Dependent variable: HbAlc

Source	Sum of type III edges	ddl	Medium square	F	Meaning	Partial sta-carr e
Corrected model	98,419.	11	8,947	3,102	,001	,126
Constant	8905,419	1	8905,419	3087,277	,000	,929
Ancdiab	60,037	3	20,012	6,938	,000	,081
Obad	4,905	2	2,452	,850	,429	,007
Ancdiab * Obad	21,592	6	3,599	1,248	,283	,031
Error	680,755	236	2,885			
Total	15344,820	248				
Total corrigd	779,173	247				

a. R-two = .126 (adjusted R-two = .086)

Tests for between-subjects effects

Dependent variable: HbAlc

Source	Sum of type III edges	ddl	Medium square	F	Meaning
Corrected model	29,371.5		5,874	1,618	,160
Constant	7271,260	1	7271,260	2003,127	,000
Old	20,870	2	10,435	2,875	,060
Tourtaille	,177	1	,177	,049	,826
Former * Tourtaille	9,080	2	4,540	1,251	,290
Error	439,224	121	3,630		
Total	8287,590	127			
Total adjusted	468,596	126			

a. R-two = .063 (adjusted R-two = .024)

Redo the analysis without the interaction term

Choose Model - Customise - Main effects.

Tests for between-subjects effects

Dependent variable: HbAlc

Source	Top of type III edges	ddl	Medium square	F	Significatio n	Partial star
Corrected model	76,827.	5	15,365	5,294	,000	,099
Constant	10183,987	1	10183,987	3508,986	,000	,935
Ancdiab	67,181	3	22,394	7,716	,000	,087

Obad	9,710	2	4,855	1,673	,190	,014
Error	702,347	242	2,902			
Total	15344,820	248				
Total adjusted	779,173	247				

a. R-two = .099 (adjusted R-two = .080)

Mean HbAlc levels: the mean HbAlc levels differed significantly according to the type of diabetes (p < 0.05), and did not differ significantly according to the age of diabetes.

6. Post hoc test

Slide old- Scheffe test :

Multiple comparisons :

Dependent variable: HbAlc

Scheffe

(I) Ancdiab	(J) Ancdiab	Average difference (I-J)	Standard error	Meaning	95% confidence interval	
					Lower terminal	Top terminal
1	2	-,596	,2738	,195	-1,367	,175
	3	-1,311*	,2738	,000	-2,082	-,540
	4	-,602	,4079	,537	-1,751	,546
2	1	,596	,2738	,195	-,175	1,367
	3	-,715	,3060	,145	-1,576	,147
	4	-,006	,4301	1,000	-1,217	1,205
3	1	1,311*	,2738	,000	,540	2,082
	2	,715	,3060	,145	-,147	1,576
	4	,709	,4301	,439	-,502	1,920
4	1	,602	,4079	,537	-,546	1,751
	2	,006	,4301	1,000	-1,205	1,217
	3	-,709	,4301	,439	-1,920	,502

Calculation based on observed averages.

The error term is the mean edge (Error) = 2.902.

*. The mean difference is significant at the .05 level.

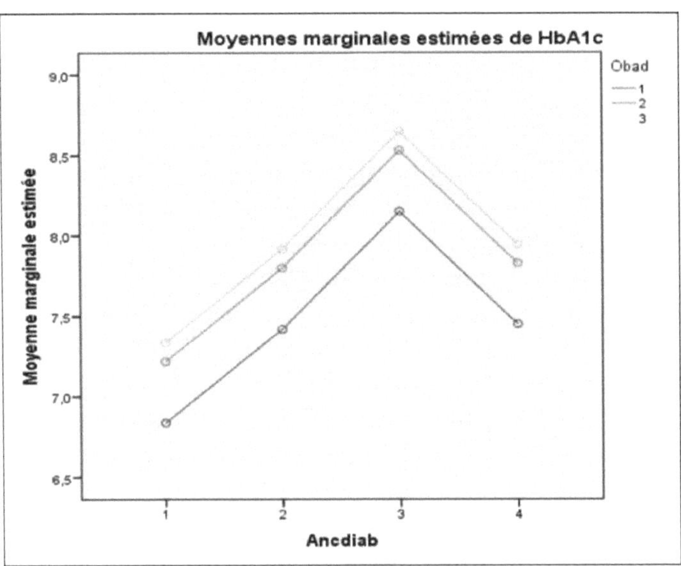

Post hoc test to find out whether these differences are due to which sub-group of the variable age, in this case it's more likely to be the code 3 modality with the highest average Hblac.

Bibliography

1) Social Statistics with IBM SPSS MD: Workbook N.E. Louis Imbeau 2017

2) Multi-variate analysis with SPSS JEAN STAFFORD PAUL BODSON

3) Precis d'epidemiologie -BEZZAOUCHA .A

4) How to perform a multivariate analysis (examples) - Selim Dahmani

5) Statistical Data Analysis with SPSS: a practical approach From comparative analyses to multiple predictive models- Sebastian Pentea,

6) Statistical processing of survey data -G Ritschard

7) Data analysis with SPSS. Cours - QCM - Exercices - Corriges. Simon Porcher, OUIDADE Sabri, Marie-Eve Laporte. August 2018

8) Principal Component Analysis with SPSS for Windows D DESBOIS 9) Data analysis with SPSS by Simon PORCHER , 10)SPSS commands associated with statistical tools- B GOVAERTS - 2016 11)L'Analyse multi variee avec SPSS. Stafford, Jean.

12) Statistical analysis and validation of a questionnaire - C Beaudart - 2021

13) Factorial Analysis And Fidelity Analysis-Claire Durant

14) Exploratory factor analysis and component analysis -JL Berger

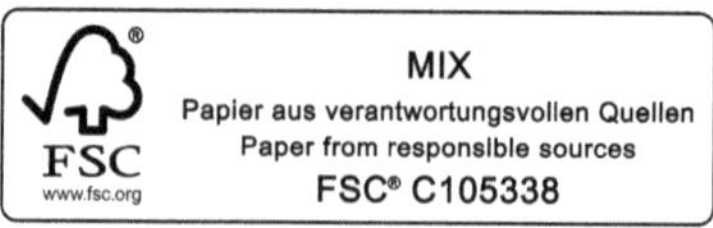

Printed by Books on Demand GmbH, Norderstedt / Germany